Chronic Diarrhea

Guest Editor

HEINZ F. HAMMER, MD

GASTROENTEROLOGY CLINICS OF NORTH AMERICA

www.gastro.theclinics.com

September 2012 • Volume 41 • Number 3

SAUNDERS an imprint of ELSEVIER, Inc.

W.B. SAUNDERS COMPANY

A Division of Elsevier Inc.

Elsevier Inc. ● 1600 John F. Kennedy Blvd., Suite 1800 ● Philadelphia, Pennsylvania 19103-2899

http://www.theclinics.com

GASTROENTEROLOGY CLINICS OF NORTH AMERICA Volume 41, Number 3
September 2012 ISSN 0889-8553, ISBN-13: 978-1-4557-3864-9

Editor: Kerry Holland
Developmental Editor: Donald Mumford

Gastroenterology Clinics of North America (ISSN 0889-8553) is published quarterly by Elsevier Inc., 360 Park Avenue South, New York, NY 10010-1710. Months of issue are March, June, September, and December. Business and Editorial Offices: 1600 John F. Kennedy Blvd., Suite 1800, Philadelphia, PA 19103-2899. Customer Service Office: 6277 Sea Harbor Drive, Orlando, FL 32887-4800. Periodicals postage paid at New York, NY and additional mailing offices. Subscription prices are $305.00 per year (US individuals), $153.00 per year (US students), $488.00 per year (US institutions), $335.00 per year (Canadian individuals), $594.00 per year (Canadian institutions), $423.00 per year (international individuals), $211.00 per year (international students), and $594.00 per year (international institutions). Foreign air speed delivery is included in all *Clinics* subscription prices. All prices are subject to change without notice. **POSTMASTER**: Send address changes to *Gastroenterology Clinics of North America*, Elsevier Health Sciences Division, Subscription Customer Service, 3251 Riverport Lane, Maryland Heights, MO 63043. Telephone: 1-800-654-2452 (U.S. and Canada); 314-447-8871 (outside U.S. and Canada). Fax: 314-447-8029. E-mail: journalscustomerservice-usa@elsevier.com (for print support); journalsonlinesupport-usa@elsevier.com (for online support).

Reprints. For copies of 100 or more, of articles in this publication, please contact the Commercial Reprints Department, Elsevier Inc., 360 Part Avenue South, New York, New York 10010-1710. Tel. (212) 633-3813, Fax: (212) 462-1935, E-mail: reprints@elsevier.com.

Gastroenterology Clinics of North America is also published in Italian by Il Pensiero Scientifico Editore, Rome, Italy; and in Portuguese by Interlivros Edicoes Ltda., Rua Commandante Coelho 1085, 21250 Cordovil, Rio de Janeiro, Brazil.

Gastroenterology Clinics of North America is covered in *MEDLINE/PubMed (Index Medicus)*, *Excerpta Medica*, *Current Contents/Clinical Medicine*, *Science Citation Index*, *ISI/BIOMED*, and *BIOSIS*.

Printed and bound by CPI Group (UK) Ltd, Croydon, CR0 4YY

Transferred to Digital Print 2012

Contributors

GUEST EDITOR

HEINZ F. HAMMER, MD
Associate Professor of Internal Medicine and Gastroenterology, Division of Gastroenterology and Hepatology, Department of Internal Medicine, Medical University of Graz, Graz, Austria; Director, Privatklinik Kastanienhof, Graz, Austria

AUTHORS

JASON A. COLE, BS
Division of Gastroenterology, Department of Internal Medicine, Baylor University Medical Center, Dallas, Texas

KATE E. EVANS, MRCP
Department of Gastroenterology and Liver Unit, Royal Hallamshire Hospital, Sheffield, South Yorkshire, United Kingdom

ELISABETH FABIAN, PhD
Division of Gastroenterology and Hepatology, Department of Internal Medicine, Medical University of Graz, Graz, Austria

JOHN S. FORDTRAN, MD
Division of Gastroenterology, Department of Internal Medicine, Baylor University Medical Center, Dallas, Texas

FABRIZIO FORTE, MD
Division of Internal Medicine and Gastroenterology, Policlinico A. Gemelli Hospital - Catholic University of Rome, Rome, Italy

ANTONIO GASBARRINI, MD
Professor of Gastroenterology, Division of Internal Medicine and Gastroenterology, Policlinico A. Gemelli Hospital - Catholic University of Rome, Rome, Italy

HEINZ F. HAMMER, MD
Associate Professor of Internal Medicine and Gastroenterology, Division of Gastroenterology and Hepatology, Department of Internal Medicine, Medical University of Graz, Graz, Austria; Director, Privatklinik Kastanienhof, Graz, Austria

JOHANN HAMMER, MD
Associate Professor of Internal Medicine and Gastroenterology, Division of Gastroenterology and Hepatology, Department of Internal Medicine, Medical University of Vienna, Vienna, Austria

CHRISTOPH HÖGENAUER, MD
Associate Professor of Medicine, Division of Gastroenterology and Hepatology, Department of Internal Medicine, Medical University of Graz, Graz, Austria

GUENTER J. KREJS, MD, AGAF
Professor of Medicine, Chief, Division of Gastroenterology and Hepatology, Department of Internal Medicine, Medical University of Graz, Graz, Austria

ELISABETH KRONES, MD
Resident in Internal Medicine, Division of Gastroenterology and Hepatology, Department of Internal Medicine, Medical University of Graz, Graz, Austria

PATRIZIA KUMP, MD
Division of Gastroenterology and Hepatology, Department of Internal Medicine, Medical University of Graz, Graz, Austria

CORD LANGNER, MD
Institute of Pathology, Medical University of Graz, Graz, Austria

SILVIA PECERE, MD
Division of Internal Medicine and Gastroenterology, Policlinico A. Gemelli Hospital - Catholic University of Rome, Rome, Italy

MARCO PIZZOFERRATO, MD
Division of Internal Medicine and Gastroenterology, Policlinico A. Gemelli Hospital - Catholic University of Rome, Rome, Italy

DAVID S. SANDERS, FACG
Department of Gastroenterology and Liver Unit, Royal Hallamshire Hospital; University of Sheffield, Sheffield, South Yorkshire, United Kingdom

CAROL A. SANTA ANA, BS
Division of Gastroenterology, Department of Internal Medicine, Baylor University Medical Center, Dallas, Texas

FRANCO SCALDAFERRI, MD
Division of Internal Medicine and Gastroenterology, Policlinico A. Gemelli Hospital - Catholic University of Rome, Rome, Italy

KAREN J. STEFFER, MD
Division of Gastroenterology, Department of Internal Medicine, Baylor University Medical Center, Dallas, Texas

JAN TACK, MD, PhD
Translational Research Center for Gastrointestinal Disorders (TARGID), University of Leuven, Leuven, Belgium

HEIMO H. WENZL, MD
Associate Professor of Medicine, Division of Gastroenterology and Hepatology, Department of Internal Medicine, Medical University of Graz, Graz, Austria

Contents

Preface: Chronic Diarrheal Disorders   ix

Heinz F. Hammer

**The Practical Value of Comprehensive Stool Analysis in Detecting the Cause
of Idiopathic Chronic Diarrhea**   539

Karen J. Steffer, Carol A. Santa Ana, Jason A. Cole, and John S. Fordtran

> The practical diagnostic value of fecal analysis in the evaluation of patients
> with chronic nonbloody diarrhea is controversial. It is possible that varia-
> tions in its value depend on how it is done and how the results are inter-
> preted rather than on its intrinsic value. In the authors' city, stool analysis
> has been made easily accessible, with a commitment to quality assurance
> and interpretation. To evaluate its practical value, the results of stool anal-
> ysis obtained on stool specimens submitted by gastroenterologists were
> retrospectively reviewed. The results indicate that stool analysis has sub-
> stantial practical diagnostic value in patients with chronic diarrhea.

**Colorectal Normal Histology and Histopathologic Findings in Patients with
Chronic Diarrhea**   561

Cord Langner

> Collagenous and lymphocytic colitis are common causes of chronic wa-
> tery diarrhea that are characterized by distinct histopathologic abnormal-
> ities without endoscopically visible lesions and are summarized as
> microscopic colitis. Several variants of microscopic colitis have been
> described, although their clinical significance still has to be defined. Pre-
> served mucosal architecture is a histologic hallmark of microscopic colitis
> and distinguishes the disease from inflammatory bowel disease (IBD). In
> addition to architectural abnormalities, the diagnosis of IBD rests on char-
> acteristic inflammatory changes. Differential diagnosis of IBD mainly in-
> cludes prolonged infection and diverticular disease–associated colitis,
> also known as segmental colitis associated with diverticulosis.

Bacterial Flora as a Cause or Treatment of Chronic Diarrhea   581

Franco Scaldaferri, Marco Pizzoferrato, Silvia Pecere, Fabrizio Forte,
and Antonio Gasbarrini

> Intestinal microflora can be considered an organ of the body. It has
> several functions in the human gut, mostly metabolic and immunologic,
> and constantly interacts with the intestinal mucosa in a delicate equilib-
> rium. Chronic diarrhea is associated with an alteration of gut microbiota
> when a pathogen invades the gut and also in several conditions asso-
> ciated with intestinal mucosal damage or bowel dysfunction, as in in-
> flammatory bowel disease, irritable bowel syndrome, or small bowel
> bacterial overgrowth. This article discusses the basis of gut microbiota
> modulation. Evidence for the efficacy of gut microbiota modulation in
> chronic conditions is also discussed.

Diarrhea Caused By Circulating Agents   603

Elisabeth Fabian, Patrizia Kump, and Guenter J. Krejs

Circulating agents cause intestinal secretion or changes in motility with decreased intestinal transit time, resulting in secretory-type diarrhea. Secretory diarrhea as opposed to osmotic diarrhea is characterized by large-volume, watery stools, often more than 1 L per day; by persistence of diarrhea when patients fast; and by the fact that on analysis of stool-water, measured osmolarity is identical to that calculated from the electrolytes present. Although sodium plays the main role in water and electrolyte absorption, chloride is the major ion involved in secretion.

Diarrhea Caused By Carbohydrate Malabsorption   611

Heinz F. Hammer and Johann Hammer

This article will focus on the role of the colon in the pathogenesis of diarrhea in carbohydrate malabsorption or physiologically incomplete absorption of carbohydrates, and on the most common manifestation of carbohydrate malabsorption, lactose malabsorption. In addition, incomplete fructose absorption, the role of carbohydrate malabsorption in other malabsorptive diseases, and congenital defects that lead to malabsorption will be covered. The article concludes with a section on diagnostic tools to evaluate carbohydrate malabsorption.

Functional Diarrhea   629

Jan Tack

Chronic diarrhea is a frequent and challenging problem in clinical medicine. In a considerable subgroup of these, no underlying cause is identified and this is referred to as functional diarrhea. A consensus definition for functional diarrhea is based on loose stool consistency and chronicity and absence of coexisting irritable bowel syndrome. Underlying pathophysiology includes rapid intestinal transit, which may be worsened by stress or be triggered by a preceding infectious gastroenteritis. Diagnostic work-up aims at exclusion of underlying organic disease. Treatment starts with dietary adjustments, aiming at decreasing nutrients that enhance transit and stool and at identifying precipitating food items.

Celiac Disease   639

Kate E. Evans and David S. Sanders

Celiac disease is common, affecting approximately 1 in 100 people, yet it remains underdiagnosed. This article reviews our current understanding of celiac disease, diagnosis, and common pitfalls. Although the cornerstone of treatment is a gluten-free diet, some patients may still have persisting symptoms and warrant further investigations.

Diarrhea in Chronic Inflammatory Bowel Diseases   651

Heimo H. Wenzl

Diarrhea is a common clinical feature of inflammatory bowel diseases and may be accompanied by abdominal pain, urgency, and fecal incontinence.

The pathophysiology of diarrhea in these diseases is complex, but defective absorption of salt and water by the inflamed bowel is the most important mechanism involved. In addition to inflammation secondary to the disease, diarrhea may arise from a variety of other conditions. It is important to differentiate the pathophysiologic mechanisms involved in the diarrhea in the individual patient to provide the appropriate therapy. This article reviews microscopic colitis, ulcerative colitis, and Crohn's disease, focusing on diarrhea.

Diarrhea in the Immunocompromised Patient 677

Elisabeth Krones and Christoph Högenauer

Diarrhea is a common problem in patients with immunocompromising conditions. The etiologic spectrum differs from patients with diarrhea who have a normal immune system. This article reviews the most important causes of diarrhea in immunocompromised patients, ranging from infectious causes to noninfectious causes of diarrhea in the setting of HIV infection as a model for other conditions of immunosuppression. It also deals with diarrhea in specific situations, eg, after hematopoietic stem cell or solid organ transplantation, diarrhea induced by immunosuppressive drugs, and diarrhea in congenital immunodeficiency syndromes.

Index 703

GASTROENTEROLOGY
CLINICS OF NORTH AMERICA

FORTHCOMING ISSUES

December 2012
Clinical Applications of Probiotics in
Gastroenterology: Questions and Answers
Gerald Friedman, MD, *Guest Editor*

March 2013
Esophageal Diseases
Nicholas Shaheen, MD, *Guest Editor*

June 2013
Gastric Cancer
Steven Moss, MD, *Guest Editor*

RECENT ISSUES

June 2012
Evaluation of Inflammatory Bowel Disease
Samir A. Shah, MD, Adam Harris, MD and
Edward Feller, MD, *Guest Editors*

March 2012
Modern Management of Benign and
Malignant Pancreatic Disease
Jacques Van Dam, MD, PhD, *Guest Editor*

December 2011
Motility Consultation: Challenges in
Gastrointestinal Motility in Everyday Clinical
Practice
Eammon M.M. Quigley, MD, *Guest Editor*

RELATED INTEREST

Emergency Medicine Clinics of North America May 2011 (Volume 29, Issue 2)
Gastrointestinal Emergencies
Angela M. Mills and Anthony J. Dean, *Guest Editors*

NOW AVAILABLE FOR YOUR iPhone and iPad

Preface
Chronic Diarrheal Disorders

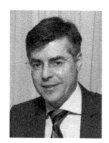

Heinz F. Hammer, MD
Guest Editor

Chronic diarrhea is defined as more than 3 bowel movements, or loose stools, for at least 4 weeks. Population-based studies from the Mayo Clinic published by Talley in 1991 have suggested a prevalence of chronic diarrhea in the United States between 14% and 18%. Features that may accompany chronic diarrhea include urgency and abdominal pain or cramps with bowel movements. A number of conditions may be responsible for chronic diarrhea, including inflammatory, neoplastic, malabsorptive, infective, and functional gastrointestinal diseases. Other causes include food intolerances, side effects of drugs, like NSAIDs, or postsurgical conditions. Diarrhea may also be a symptom of a systemic disease, like diabetes or hyperthyroidism. Special patient groups, like the very elderly and patients in the intensive care unit, pose special challenges in the diagnosis and treatment of chronic diarrhea.

Chronic diarrhea may result in a multitude of clinical and social problems for patients. In a small minority of patients chronic diarrhea is the main symptom and can be life threatening, due to excessive fluid and electrolyte losses, for example, in some endocrine tumors. In a considerably larger proportion of patients chronic diarrhea is part of a symptom complex, like in inflammatory bowel diseases, and in these patients other symptoms, like blood loss or abdominal pain, may have more clinical relevance than diarrhea. However, the most frequent causes of diarrhea are functional and have neither life-threatening consequences nor are they a sign of a severe underlying disease, although also in these patients chronic diarrhea may severely inflict on quality of life, due to the interference of diarrhea, fecal urgency, or fecal incontinence with normal professional or social daily activities.

The topics selected for this issue of *Gastroenterology Clinics of North America* reach beyond knowledge that can be easily obtained from the standard gastroenterology textbooks. They rather focus on specific topics and present in-depth reviews on specific issues in the diagnostic evaluation and pathophysiology of chronic diarrheal disorders. The issue starts with an article on the practical value of stool analysis in detecting the etiology of idiopathic chronic diarrhea. The authors of this article have complemented their large experience by recent research. This is followed by an article

Gastroenterol Clin N Am 41 (2012) ix–x
http://dx.doi.org/10.1016/j.gtc.2012.07.001
0889-8553/12/$ – see front matter © 2012 Elsevier Inc. All rights reserved.

gastro.theclinics.com

that thoroughly describes normal colorectal histology and, based on this knowledge, extends to histopathologic findings in patients with chronic diarrhea. The recent interest in the role of the bacterial flora as a cause or treatment of chronic diarrhea is discussed in the third article. This is followed by an article summarizing the role of circulating agents in the pathogenesis of diarrhea and by articles on some specific conditions or disorders causing diarrhea, that is, diarrhea in carbohydrate malabsorption, functional diarrhea, celiac disease, inflammatory bowel diseases, and diarrhea in the immunocompromised host.

I am confident that this issue offers the most current information regarding this important condition and I am grateful to the authors that they have focused on information that can be taken to the bedside and immediately applied.

Heinz F. Hammer, MD
Med. University of Graz
Auenbruggerplatz 15
8036 Graz, Austria

E-mail address:
heinz.hammer@medunigraz.at

The Practical Value of Comprehensive Stool Analysis in Detecting the Cause of Idiopathic Chronic Diarrhea

Karen J. Steffer, MD, Carol A. Santa Ana, BS, Jason A. Cole, BS, John S. Fordtran, MD*

KEYWORDS

- Stool analysis • Fecal electrolytes • Diarrhea • Secretory diarrhea • Steatorrhea
- Carbohydrate malabsorption • Functional diarrhea • Laxative induced diarrhea

KEY POINTS

- The practical diagnostic value of fecal analysis in the evaluation of patients with idiopathic chronic non-bloody diarrhea is controversial due to questions related to its unpleasant nature, quality control, interpretation of results, and intrinsic value.
- To evaluate its diagnostic value we retrospectively reviewed the results obtained on 158 stool specimens that were submitted by orders of practicing gastroenterologists during an 18 month period.
- A specific cause of chronic diarrhea was identified in 8% of cases; in addition, steatorrhea was found in 28%, and probable carbohydrate malabsorption without steatorrhea in 18% of cases.
- Positive findings were almost as frequent in patients with stool weights less than 200 g/d as in patients with stool weights greater than 200 g/d.
- In the authors' opinion, these results indicate that stool analysis has substantial practical diagnostic value in patients with idiopathic chronic diarrhea.

INTRODUCTION

In a substantial fraction of patients with chronic nonbloody diarrhea, the cause is not apparent from the history, physical examination, routine laboratory data, or from a search for an infectious organism. In the United States, such patients often

Supported by the Southwest Digestive Disease Foundation and by Baylor Healthcare System Foundation.

Division of Gastroenterology, Department of Internal Medicine, Baylor University Medical Center, 3500 Gaston Avenue, Dallas, TX 75246, USA

* Corresponding author.

E-mail address: JohnFO@BaylorHealth.edu

Gastroenterol Clin N Am 41 (2012) 539–560

http://dx.doi.org/10.1016/j.gtc.2012.06.001

0889-8553/12/$ – see front matter © 2012 Elsevier Inc. All rights reserved.

undergo exhaustive diagnostic studies, including colonoscopy with mucosal biopsies; upper endoscopy with duodenal biopsy; computed tomography (CT) scan of the abdomen and pelvis; small bowel evaluation by camera, endoscopy, or CT; octreotide scan; and the measurement of plasma peptides. Additional tests can include celiac disease antibody panel, a search for unusual pathogenic microorganisms, culture of jejunal fluid for anaerobic bacterial overgrowth, measurement of serotonin metabolites, and measurement of fecal bile acids. However, in many patients, a specific cause cannot be identified even after they have been subjected to most or all of these tests. The causes of diarrhea that escape detection by these methods include inadvertent or surreptitious laxative ingestion; excess consumption of poorly absorbed carbohydrates; several causes of undetected malabsorption; undiagnosed or undiagnosable infections; alterations in colonic bacterial flora[1]; autonomic neuropathy causing rapid transit; thyrotoxicosis and other endocrinopathies; immune reactions to food; adverse reaction to medications, food additives, or supplements; and anatomic changes in the pelvic floor or anal sphincter that produce fecal incontinence.

The fraction of patients with idiopathic chronic diarrhea who remain undiagnosed is highly variable depending on criteria for patient selection. The undiagnosed fraction will also vary depending on the diagnostic definitions applied. For example, some physicians make a diagnosis of irritable bowel syndrome or functional diarrhea when preliminary tests are negative and stool weight is estimated to be low or measured to be less than 200 g/d. The authors do not do this because they know of no evidence showing that stool weight less than 200 g/d excludes organic causes of diarrhea. Thus, the undiagnosed fraction according to the authors' definitions would be higher.

In addition to the fact that current strategies often fail to reveal a specific cause of idiopathic chronic diarrhea,[2–4] the costs of diagnostic tests and procedures are considerable. Therefore, in the opinion of some clinical investigators in the United States, the early phase of evaluation should include a stool analysis that measures fecal weight, fecal fat output, and fecal fluid electrolyte concentrations.[5–7] Such analysis can classify chronic diarrhea into different pathophysiological categories, which helps select diagnostic procedures that are most likely to reveal the underlying cause and reduce the use of unnecessary procedures. In addition, stool analysis can identify patients who are surreptitiously or inadvertently ingesting osmotic laxatives.

Although the logic for using comprehensive stool analysis in patients with chronic diarrhea seems sound, such testing is not readily accessible in most clinical centers in the United States. Various components of the analysis must be ordered individually from reference laboratories, and the results are reported without an overall interpretation. As a result, comprehensive stool analysis is rarely used. This situation may not be a big loss because in the United Kingdom, the measurement of fecal fat and fecal fluid electrolytes is considered to have little practical value in patients with chronic diarrhea.[8–10] This negative opinion seems to be based on the inconvenience and unpleasant nature of collecting and analyzing stool specimens, lack of quality control, and problems related to the interpretation of the results. It is possible that this negative view was also influenced by data showing that, in general practice, stool analysis is inherently unable to provide results that are diagnostically useful; if such data exist, the authors are not aware of it.

The authors accept the view that if analytical procedures are not accurately performed, and if results are not properly interpreted, stool analysis would have little practical value in detecting the cause of idiopathic chronic diarrhea. However, the authors think there is another reasonable question to ask. If stool analysis were accurately performed and interpreted, would it then have practical value?

PRESENT STUDY

About 25 years ago, Baylor University Medical Center established a laboratory to facilitate the evaluation of patients with chronic diarrhea. The laboratory is under the administrative direction of the gastroenterology department, and quality assurance is monitored by a third-party accreditation agency, Commission of Office Laboratory Accreditation (COLA). One of this laboratory's missions is to perform and interpret a defined panel of analytical tests on stool specimens collected from patients with chronic diarrhea. Many practicing gastroenterologists in the Dallas area now use this laboratory in the evaluation of their private patients. A recent survey of these gastroenterologists revealed that most consider stool analysis as completing a diagnostic workup rather than as a guide for cost-effective utilization of other diagnostic procedures. They usually request stool analysis after endoscopic procedures and biopsies have failed to reveal a diagnosis. These gastroenterologists think that comprehensive stool analysis is extremely useful to them and to their patients.

In an effort to gain insight into the practical diagnostic value of comprehensive stool analysis in adult patients with chronic diarrhea, the authors retrospectively studied results obtained on 158 stool specimens that were submitted by orders of practicing gastroenterologists during the 18-month period between January 1, 2010 and June 30, 2011. This study was performed without knowledge of other diagnostic tests that had been performed or the cause of diarrhea that may have been ultimately discovered. It was approved by the institutional review board of Baylor Research Institute.

STOOL COLLECTION, METHODS OF ANALYSIS, AND INTERPRETATION

When stool collections were done at home, patients were instructed to collect stools quantitatively for a defined period of time and to continue to eat their regular diet during the collection period. Along with verbal and written instructions, they were provided with a Styrofoam (Dow Chemical Company, Midland, Michigan) cooler, ice packs, a collection device, and containers for storing stool during the collection period. Using the provided equipment, the temperature in the cooler ranges from 4°C to 10°C.[11] The time of the stool collection was 24, 48, or 72 hours, as specified by the referring physician. During the collection period, patients were instructed to record food intake, the time of each bowel movement, and note if any stool was not collected. Patients were asked to deliver their collected stool specimen to the laboratory as soon as possible after the timed collection was complete. When stools were collected in the hospital, the same protocol was used except that stools specimens were stored in a portable refrigerator and, on completion, they were returned to the laboratory by the nursing staff.

Specimens from 32 patients were not included in the present study of 158 patients for the following reasons: 11 reported incomplete stool collections; for 8, the referring physician noted previous intestinal surgery, which would probably be the cause of their diarrhea; in 5 specimens, the technician detected urine contamination; 3 collected their specimen while fasting; 3 had missing or incomplete data; and in 2, specimens were collected on more than one occasion and only the first was included.

On receipt of the specimen, stool consistency was graded. Stools were then weighed and homogenized. A sample of the homogenized stool was analyzed for fat concentration by the van de Kamer method.[12] Fecal fat output (grams per day) was calculated by multiplying the fecal fat concentration by stool weight. When fat output was greater than 7.0 g/d, the stool was analyzed for chymotrypsin activity.[13] The homogenized stool specimen was also analyzed for excess fecal neutrophils by the Wampole Leuko Ez Vue method for lactoferrin and for occult blood by Hemoccult II. Another sample of the homogenized stool was centrifuged (25,000 rpm for 1 hour), and the fecal supernatant was analyzed for sodium and potassium by Jenway PFP7/C flame photometer (Essex, England), for chloride by Labconco chloride analyzer (Labconco, Kansas City, Missouri), for bicarbonate by Corning 965 carbon dioxide analyzer (Essex, England), for pH by Radiometer PHM 82 Standard pH meter (Radiometer America Inc, Westlake, Ohio), and for osmolality by freezing point depression (Micro-Osmometer model 3MO; Advanced Instruments, Norwood, Massachusetts).

The results were written on a report form and then interpreted by one of the authors (JSF) without knowledge of the patient's medical history or other diagnostic tests that had been performed. The interpreter sometimes recommended further analytical studies on the stool specimens. The report form was faxed to the referring physician within a few days of receipt of the specimen. The form the authors use, as well as the results and interpretation of one highly selected and dramatic case from the present series of patients, are shown in **Fig. 1**.

In this article, the authors do not present or discuss results on occult blood, chymotrypsin activity, or lactoferrin. Their inclusion would have required many additional subdivisions that would obscure the primary objective of evaluating fecal weight, fecal fat, and fecal fluid electrolyte concentrations.

DEFINITIONS
Objective Evidence of Diarrhea

Stool consistency was graded according to the following scale: (1) formed, firm; (2) formed, soft; (3) unformed, soft; (4) unformed, mushy; (5) runny; (6) watery. Grades 1 and 2 were considered normal consistency and grades 3 to 6 were considered abnormal.

An abnormal increase in bowel movement frequency was defined as more than 3 bowel movements per day. Hyperdefecation was defined as 4 or more bowel movements per day when stool weight was less than 200 g/d. The authors do not use the term hyperdefecation when stool weight exceeds 200 g/d. Objective evidence of diarrhea was considered to be present when 1 or more of the following criteria were met: (1) consistency graded greater than or equal to 3, as described earlier; (2) stool weight greater than 200 g/d; and (3) average bowel movement frequency greater than 3 times per day.

Steatorrhea

The upper limit for fecal fat output in healthy patients ingesting their normal diet is approximately 7 g/d when measured by the van de Kamer method.[4] However, healthy patients with diarrhea induced by laxatives can have fecal fat outputs as high as 14 g/d, despite maintaining their normal diets.[14] Thus, even when intake, digestion, and absorption of dietary fat are normal, diarrhea per se can cause a secondary steatorrhea, with fecal fat outputs as high as 14 g/d. Therefore, in patients with diarrhea, fecal fat output between 7 and 14 g/d will have a low specificity for identifying primary defects in fat digestion or absorption. Based on the progressive increase in fecal fat output as stool weight increases,[14] the authors defined fat malabsorption in patients with chronic diarrhea as follows: stool weight up to 400 g/d, fecal fat output greater than 7 g/d; stool weight 400 to 1000 g/d, fecal fat output greater than 11 g/d; stool

Fecal Analysis
G.I. Analytical Laboratory
Baylor University Medical Center, Dallas, TX

Patient name: -----   Age/Sex: -----
Doctor: -----   Case No.: -----

Length of Collection: 24 (eating) hours
Fecal Weight (nl <200 g/day): 3745 g/day
 # Bowel Movements/day: 20
Fecal Consistency: Watery

Fecal Consistency Grading:	
1 – Formed, firm	4 – Unformed, mushy
2 – Formed, soft	5 – Runny
3 – Unformed, soft	6 – Watery

Chemical Analysis:

Osmolality	281 mOsm/kg	**Osmotic Gap:** -52 [= 290 – 2([Na]+[K])]
pH	6.60	
[Na]	158 mEq/L	**Anion Gap:** 159 [=([Na]+[K])-([Cl]+[HCO₃])]
[K]	13 mEq/L	
[Cl]	8 mEq/L	
[HCO₃]	4 mEq/L	

Qualitative Reducing Substances: -----

Hemoccult II (Test for blood): Negative

Fecal Lactoferrin (Test for fecal neutrophils): Negative

Fecal Fat Analysis:
    Concentration: 0.06 g / 100g stool
    Output (nl <7 g/day):   2.2 g/day

Interpretation:
Extremely severe diarrhea, with Na and K concentration approaching the concentration of these cations in plasma. This is reminiscent of fecal electrolyte output in cholera. However, the fecal Cl concentration is very low, and the osmotic gap is negative. Although the significance of low Cl and negative osmotic gap in this case are unclear, these are features that have been observed in patients who have high fecal concentrations of a divalent anion. There is no evidence of bleeding, excess fecal neutrophils, or steatorrhea. The stool sample was labeled as being collected when the patient was eating.

Addendum:
    Phosphate   117 mmol/L (438 mmol/day)
        Interpretation: The fecal fluid concentration and daily output of phosphate are extremely high, suggesting that the patient is ingesting very large amounts of phosphate, and that this is causing her severe diarrhea. Excess phosphate ingestion causes diarrhea that appears to be secretory in type, but is actually osmotic diarrhea with a negative osmotic gap.

    Sulfate   2.60 mmol/L (9.7 mmol/day)

Fig. 1. An example of report form and interpretation that are generated from stool analysis and sent to the referring physician.

weight greater than 1000 g/d fecal fat output greater than 14 g/d. The authors have no data on fecal fat output by healthy patients with laxative-induced diarrhea who have stool weights greater than 1800 g/d. Nevertheless, in the authors' laboratory, patients with extreme diarrhea (2000–4000 g/d) are considered to have fat malabsorption only if their fecal fat output exceeds 16 g/d.

    Dietary fat intake in the patients was unknown. Patients were not asked to change their diet to standardize fat intake because it takes at least 1 week to develop a new steady state and because actual fat intake would remain unknown. If fat intake in a patient was low, fecal fat output might be within normal limits in a patient who has fat malabsorption. However, in patients with fat malabsorption caused by nontropical sprue, Comfort and colleagues found that fecal fat output on a diet containing about 50 g/d of fat exceeded the upper limit of normal obtained with a test diet that contained approximately twice as much fat.[15] If fat intake was very high, it might cause spurious steatorrhea, although the magnitude of excess fecal fat would probably be trivial because when normal people ingested 30, 60, 100, and 200 g/d of fat, average fecal fat output was 3.2, 4.0, 4.8, and 7.8 g/d, respectively.[16] Based on these considerations, the authors think fecal fat output has diagnostic value even when fecal fat intake is unknown. Obviously, the interpretation of fecal fat output would be more accurate if dietary fat were known and taken into account. The accuracy of daily fecal fat measurement is also limited by the short collection periods (1–3 days). The errors induced by short collection periods are probably less in patients with either voluminous diarrhea or increased bowel movement frequency than in healthy subjects without diarrhea.

Distinguishing Secretory from Osmotic Diarrhea

As explained elsewhere,[4,17] fluid in the colon and rectum is equilibrated with extracellular fluid within the body and its osmolality is approximately 290 mOsm/kg. The traditional way in which electrolyte and nonelectrolyte solute composition of fecal fluid is expressed is by calculation of the osmotic gap.

$$\text{Osmotic gap} = 290 - [([Na] + [K]) \times 2]$$

The sum of sodium and potassium concentrations is multiplied by 2 to account for associated, mostly monovalent anions; the result approximates the total concentration of electrolytes in fecal fluid. Even though measured osmolality is not used to calculate the osmotic gap, it is always measured to detect the dilution of the stool with extraneous water (measured as a fecal fluid osmolality less than 290 mOsm/kg).

Secretory diarrhea is caused by reduced absorption or increased intestinal secretion of electrolytes and water. In this type of diarrhea, the sum of [Na] and [K] is close to 140 mEq/L, and the osmotic gap is near zero. In osmotic diarrhea, active absorption and secretion of electrolytes are normal, but some extraneous osmotically active solute exists in intestinal fluid that prevents water absorption. In this form of diarrhea, the osmolality of fecal fluid is, to a substantial extent, made up of nonelectrolytes, and the concentration of monovalent electrolytes is correspondingly low; therefore, the osmotic gap is large.

The cutoff points for osmotic gap that distinguish secretory from osmotic diarrhea cannot be derived from a study of patients with chronic diarrhea because in most patients there is no independent way of knowing the mechanisms of their diarrhea. However, electrolyte concentrations of fecal fluid in healthy subjects with diarrhea induced by substances that produce secretory or osmotic diarrhea have been measured. From these results, cutoff values for osmotic gap, chloride concentration, and pH were found that can (1) distinguish between osmotic and secretory diarrhea and (2) suggest when magnesium, polyethylene glycol, sulfate, or phosphate is being used to produce factitious osmotic diarrhea. These results have been described in detail elsewhere.[4,18,19]

Carbohydrate Malabsorption

Unlike fat malabsorption, carbohydrate malabsorption cannot be measured simply by analyzing stools for carbohydrate content because colonic bacteria metabolize some or all of the carbohydrate that is unabsorbed by the small intestine. This fermentation takes place within the lumen of the colon and also to some extent in the collection container after stool is passed. For this reason, the amount of carbohydrate excreted in stool does not accurately reflect the amount of carbohydrate that was not absorbed. For research purposes, it is possible to measure carbohydrates and organic acids in stool and to quantitate total carbohydrate equivalents appearing in stool,[17,20] but these methods are too time consuming to incorporate into a routine clinical stool analysis panel. Stool analysis to detect carbohydrate malabsorption for clinical purposes has, therefore, depended on 2 measurements: fecal electrolyte concentrations, which are not altered by bacterial fermentation after stools have been passed, and the pH of fecal fluid. Unlike fat malabsorption, wherein output is quantitatively measured, carbohydrate malabsorption is defined only as present or absent; the accuracy of the result is not dependent on the quantitative collection of stools.

Diarrhea induced in healthy subjects by the ingestion of lactulose or sorbitol 4 times daily was almost always associated with a fecal fluid osmotic gap between 75 to 240 mOsm/kg.[17,18] This wide range of elevated gaps is mainly caused by differences in the degree to which unabsorbed sugars in colonic fluid are converted by colonic bacteria to organic acids. The colon reabsorbs a fraction of these organic acids, but unabsorbed organic acids in colonic fluid form salts by combining with sodium and potassium. When fecal fluid contains high concentrations of sodium and potassium salts of organic acids, the sodium and potassium concentrations in fecal fluid increase and the osmotic gap is low. On the other hand, when colonic fluid contains high concentrations of monosaccharides or disaccharides, the osmotic gap is high. In addition to an osmotic gap greater than 75 mOsm/kg, almost all subjects ingesting lactulose or sorbitol had a fecal fluid pH less than 5.5. In contrast, other causes of experimental diarrhea in healthy subjects were almost never associated with a fecal fluid pH less than 5.5.

Based on the results with lactulose and sorbitol, it might be expected that diarrhea produced by carbohydrate malabsorption is always associated with both a large osmotic gap and a low fecal pH. However, when patients with chronic diarrhea caused by known carbohydrate malabsorption (diagnosed by the measurement of fecal water obligated by reducing sugars, organic acids, and associated cations) were studied, only 2 of 6 patients had a fecal fluid pH less than 5.5.[4] This finding suggests that there may be a pH discrepancy between healthy subjects ingesting lactulose and sorbitol compared to patients with disorders that impair absorption of normal dietary carbohydrates.

To obtain further information on malabsorption of physiologic dietary carbohydrates, for the past 3 years the authors have studied fecal fluid from patients who develop diarrhea while undergoing a breath hydrogen test to detect lactose malabsorption. (None of the patients undergoing breath tests were part of the 158 patients with chronic diarrhea that are the main focus of this article.) The main goal was to study concordance between fecal fluid osmotic gap and pH criteria that are used for the identification of carbohydrate malabsorption. In addition to the usual tests in the stool analysis panel, the concentrations of total carbohydrate and organic acids in fecal fluid were also measured.

Table 1 shows results in 16 patients who developed diarrhea during a 3-hour period after ingesting 50 g of lactose and whose fecal fluid had either an osmotic gap greater than or equal to 75 mOsm/kg or a pH less than 5.5. Fourteen of these patients had a positive lactose breath test, whereas 2 did not. Fecal fluid osmotic gap was greater than 75 mOsm/kg in all 16 patients, whereas fecal fluid pH was less than 5.5 in only 3 patients. No patient had a low pH without an associated increased osmotic gap.

Table 1
Fecal analysis in 16 patients who developed diarrhea after ingesting 50 g of lactose

Lactose Breath Test[a] H+ (ppm)		Stool Weight Within 3 h After Lactose Load (g)	Consistency	Concentrations (mEq/L)			Osmotic Gap (mOsm/kg)	CHO (g/L)	Organic Acids (mEq/L)	pH
Baseline	Peak			Na	K	Cl				
2	21	355	Runny	49	9	32	174	20.9	24	7.20
3	92	54 (FI)	Runny	32	32	4	162	1.9	66	5.81
0	246	171	Runny	32	33	16	160	6.3	106	5.46
0	44	97	Soft	21	49	15	150	10.8	NA	5.65
3	192	48	Runny	39	32	64	148	26.2	120	5.22
0	83	319	Runny	38	35	15	144	31.3	123	5.60
2	98	103	Runny	41	33	30	142	9.0	124	5.99
11	>400	60	Soft	8	67	16	140	1.9	118	6.87
2	310	365	Watery	31	49	23	130	21.6	89	5.81
2	82	517	Watery	67	16	54	124	9.9	28	6.91
12	157	261	Runny	58	31	34	112	16.5	149	5.25
1	186	400	Runny	24	66	16	110	18.0	126	6.05
15	208	220	Runny	36	56	15	106	6.2	402	5.75
14	248	359	Runny	40	57	25	96	8.4	155	6.30
17	22	112	Soft	34	72	8	78	7.2	212	6.12
19	>400	78	Runny	64	43	45	76	6.4	129	6.88

Reference values for 25 diarrheal specimens induced with PEG (mean ± sem, range)

Stool Weight (g/24 h)	Consistency	Na	K	Cl	Osmotic Gap (mOsm/kg)	CHO (g/L)	Organic Acids (mEq/L)	pH
			(mEq/L)					
740 ± 64 (285–1417)	Runny	11.4 ± 1.5 (2.9–27.1)	13.3 ± 0.9 (6.2–22.5)	7.2 ± 0.5 (3–11)	241 ± 3 (213–267)	1.0 ± 0.1 (0.3–2.3)	64 ± 5 (30–138)	6.21 ± 0.09 (5.50–7.03)

[a] An increase of 20 ppm from baseline indicates a positive breath test for lactose malabsorption.
Abbreviation: FI, Fecal Incontinence.

Fourteen had an abnormally high fecal fluid concentration of carbohydrate compared to normal subjects with diarrhea induced by polyethylene glycol (PEG). In contrast, the concentration of organic acids in fecal fluid was elevated in only 4 of 15 patients. There was no statistically significant correlation between organic acid concentration and pH ($R = 0.33$, $P = .237$).

These fecal fluid pH results with lactose-induced diarrhea are similar to results in patients with malabsorption of dietary carbohydrate[4] but not to results obtained in healthy subjects who had diarrhea caused by ingestion of lactulose or sorbitol. In the authors' opinion, the most likely explanation for the pH discrepancy between previous studies with lactulose/sorbitol and current studies with lactose is that much less carbohydrate was malabsorbed in the lactose studies. Other investigators have discussed other factors that influence fecal fluid pH in people with carbohydrate malabsorption.[21–23]

In regard to detecting malabsorption of lactose, the authors conclude that a fecal fluid osmotic gap of greater than or equal to 75 mOsm/kg occurs much more frequently than a pH less than 5.5. The value of osmotic gap is enhanced by the fact that it does not change during storage of stool samples, regardless of storage temperature. As a confirmatory test for lactose malabsorption, measuring the concentration of carbohydrate in fecal fluid would be more useful than measuring organic acid concentration. The diagnostic value of either carbohydrate or organic acid concentrations depends on the maintenance of a cold temperature during storage.[20]

For the 158 patients in the present study, if the osmotic gap was greater than 75 mOsm/kg, it was concluded that the patient might have carbohydrate malabsorption. If further analysis did not reveal either magnesium- or PEG-induced diarrhea, the patient was considered to have probable carbohydrate malabsorption. There are several other rare but possible causes of an osmotic gap greater than or equal to 75 mOsm/kg, such as urea (fistula between gastrointestinal and genitourinary tracts), ammonium (NH_4), or amino acids. The authors have never knowingly encountered these as causes of a high osmotic gap, but in special circumstances fecal fluid is analyzed for these solutes. Independent of the osmotic gap, if the fecal fluid pH was less than 5.5, and if the fecal chloride concentration was less than 100 mEq/L to exclude congenital chloridorrhea,[23] the patient was considered to have carbohydrate malabsorption.

Magnesium-Induced Diarrhea

Magnesium-induced diarrhea is considered when fecal fluid osmotic gap exceeds 75 mOsm/kg[18] and is confirmed when fecal magnesium concentration exceeds 80 mEq/L.[24] When the magnesium concentration is between 80 and 160 mEq/L, magnesium is responsible for a substantial part of the diarrhea, but an additional cause of diarrhea is also contributing. The additional cause might include a disease process or ingestion of another laxative, such as bisacodyl or senna. When the magnesium concentration is 160 mEq/L or higher, excess magnesium ingestion is the only cause of the diarrhea.

RESULTS AND COMMENTS
Patient Demographics

Based on a survey of referring gastroenterologists, the likelihood of referral of a particular patient increased if preliminary endoscopic procedures, histopathologic analysis of biopsies, and radiologic imaging did not reveal a diagnosis. This practice would reduce the prevalence of inflammatory bowel disease, microscopic colitis, and celiac

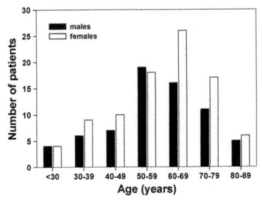

Fig. 2. Age distribution of 158 patients with chronic diarrhea who submitted stool specimens for analysis. Solid bars denote men and open bars denote women.

disease in those who were referred for comprehensive stool analysis. The likelihood of referral probably increased if patients were in advanced age groups wherein the probability of a malignancy is perceived to be increased. Suspicion of surreptitious laxative ingestion would enhance the likelihood of referral and this could result in referral of more women than men.

The specimens that the authors analyzed were collected from 158 patients who were under the care of 40 physicians. None of the patients were under the care of the authors. Seventy-seven percent of the specimens were collected from outpatients. The patients who submitted specimens were mainly between 50 and 80 years of age, and the female-to-male ratio was 1.3:1.0 (**Fig. 2**). Twenty-one percent of the patients had stool weights less than 200 g/d and 15% had stool weights greater than 1000 g/d (**Fig. 3**).

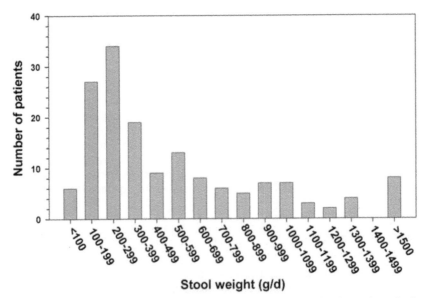

Fig. 3. Distribution of stool weights in 158 patients with chronic diarrhea who submitted stool specimens for analysis.

Pathophysiological Categories with Practical Diagnostic Value

Based on the results of stool analysis, each of the 158 patients was assigned to 1 of the 6 categories shown in **Fig. 4**. The number of men and women in each category is shown. Each patient is plotted as a function of his or her daily stool weight. The scale of the vertical axis is logarithmic to show the extreme range of stool weights in most categories. A dotted horizontal line separates patients with stool weights less than 200 g/d from those with higher stool weights.

The first 5 categories in **Fig. 4** are pathophysiological patterns from stool analysis that the authors consider to be diagnostically useful. These categories are not all of the pathophysiological categories that can be derived from stool analysis but are those the authors think have diagnostic value. For example, secretory diarrhea with steatorrhea was not included because the significance of steatorrhea is not altered by the presence or absence of secretory diarrhea. Dilution of the stools with water is a diagnostically useful pathophysiological category but it was not included because none of the specimens in this series had a measured fecal fluid osmolality substantially less than 290 mOsm/kg. The final category, **Fig. 4F**, is for patients whose stool analysis did not reveal a diagnostically useful pattern (unclassified patients). Each of the 6 categories shown in **Fig. 4** are discussed in the following paragraphs.

Patients with stool weights less than 200 g/d

As shown in **Fig. 4**A, 33 patients (21% of the total) had stool weights less than 200 g/d. Nine were men and 24 were women. Subclassifications of these 33 patients are

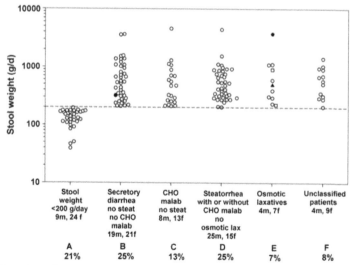

Fig. 4. Allocation of 158 patients with chronic diarrhea to 6 different categories based on stool analysis. In category B, open symbols denote classic secretory diarrhea and the closed symbol denotes a patient with potassium-mediated secretory diarrhea. In category E, the open circles represent patients with elevated fecal fluid magnesium concentrations between 80 and 160 mEq/L; the open squares represent patients that had fecal fluid magnesium concentrations exceeding 160 mEq/L; the solid circle represents a patient with phosphate-induced diarrhea, and the solid triangle represents a patient with PEG-induced diarrhea. Category F is for patients in whom stool analysis did not reveal what was considered to be a diagnostically useful pattern. The percentages shown at the bottom of the figure represents the percent of patients in each category derived from the 158 patient cohort.

Table 2
Stool analysis in 33 patients with stool weight less than 200 g/d

Category	n	Sex	Average Age (Range) (y)	Average Stool Weight (Range) (g/d)	Average BM Frequency (Range)	Average Stool Consistency (Range)	Average Fecal Fat (Range) (g/d)	Fecal Fluid Obtained (n)	Average Osmotic Gap (Range) (mOsm/kg)	Average pH (Range)
No objective evidence of diarrhea No malabsorption No laxatives	9	Male = 0 Female = 9	65 (27–88)	113 (46–172)	1.9 (1–3)	1.2 (1–2)	4.0 (1.4–6.7)	5	34 (−10 to 60)	6.89 (6.14–8.49)
Hyperdefecation No malabsorption No laxatives	6	Male = 1 Female = 5	70 (51–87)	131 (91–162)	9.8 (4–23)	3.0 (2–5)	2.5 (0.9–4.9)	6	29 (−14 to 68)	6.78 (6.25–7.59)
Unformed stools No hyperdefecation No malabsorption No laxatives	6	Male = 3 Female = 3	54 (22–77)	126 (39–175)	1.5 (1–3)	4.5 (3–5)	1.7 (0.2–4.6)	5	3 (−42 to 48)	6.37 (5.52–7.49)
High magnesium No malabsorption	1	Male = 1	51	173	1.5	2	1.8	1	200	6.47
Carbohydrate malabsorption without steatorrhea	7	Male = 1 Female = 6	53 (29–79)	153 (121–178)	2.4 (0.5–4.0)	3.4 (2–5)	2.1 (0.4–4.4)	7	87 (78 to 112)	6.67 (5.89–8.36)
Steatorrhea	4	Males = 3 Females = 1	64 (45–84)	152 (130–193)	1.2 (1.0–1.5)	1.8 (1–2)	15.9 (8.8–21.8)	2	−31 (−44 to −18)	6.63 (6.60–6.65)

provided in **Table 2**. The first row in **Table 2** shows results in 9 patients who had no objective evidence of diarrhea, no evidence of malabsorption of fat or carbohydrate, and no evidence of laxative ingestion. All of these patients were women. Despite the absence of objective evidence of diarrhea, these patients presumably considered themselves to have chronic diarrhea. Five explanations for this apparent contradiction can be suggested. First, even though stool weight, bowel movement frequency, and consistency of stools were within the limits of normal, these patients might have experienced a change in one of these objective parameters (for example, from 1 to 3 bowel movements per day). Second, their diarrhea might be intermittent or recurring rather than persistent and, hence, not present during their stool collection. Third, the patients may have altered their dietary intake during the collection period (despite instructions to continue their normal diet). Fourth, some of these patients may have been treated with an opiate antidiarrheal drug, which could have eliminated objective evidence of diarrhea. Fifth, some of these patients may have been suffering from incontinence, a symptom that many patients withhold from their physician unless they are specifically questioned.[2] When interpreting and reporting the results of stool analysis in such patients, the authors often suggest collection of a random stool sample for reanalysis if and when stools become runny.

The second row in **Table 2** shows results on 6 patients who had hyperdefecation, without evidence of malabsorption or laxative intake. Their bowel movement frequency averaged 9.8 times per day. Stool consistency was highly variable. The third row in **Table 2** shows results on 6 patients who had soft, unformed to runny stools with no hyperdefecation or evidence of malabsorption or laxative intake. In the authors' opinion, further diagnostic evaluation is warranted in the patients described in the second and third rows, directed toward disorders of the rectosigmoid colon and fecal continence mechanisms. This evaluation would include a careful rectal examination and a sigmoidoscopy with biopsies. Women in this category should have a pelvic examination and a pelvic sonogram. It may be helpful to keep in mind that patients with low-volume diarrhea and decreased stool consistency may benefit symptomatically from the use of psyllium-containing products.[25,26]

The fourth row in **Table 2** shows results on 1 male patient who had no objective evidence of diarrhea and no malabsorption but who had a fecal osmotic gap of 200 mOsm/kg and a fecal fluid magnesium concentration of 138 mEq/L. These findings indicate that magnesium increased the effective osmotic pressure of his fecal fluid and thereby reduced colonic absorption of water. The magnitude of excess magnesium intake in this patient must have been small (such as that contained in oral magnesium supplements rather than laxatives) because his average stool weight was only 173 g/d. The clinical implications of magnesium-induced diarrhea are discussed in a later section on osmotic laxatives.

The fifth row in **Table 2** shows results on 7 patients who had high fecal fluid osmotic gaps without evidence of osmotic laxative intake or steatorrhea, indicating that they had carbohydrate malabsorption. The sixth row of **Table 2** shows results on 4 patients who had steatorrhea, with an average fecal fat output of 15.9 g/d. Fecal fat concentrations in these 4 patients were 6.4, 9.0, 11.3, and 14.3 g/100 g wet stool weight. The diagnostic significance of finding carbohydrate malabsorption (row 5) and steatorrhea (row 6) are discussed in subsequent sections.

Secretory diarrhea without steatorrhea, stool weight greater than 200 g/d

For purposes of this presentation, the authors designated patients with an osmotic gap less than or equal to 50 mOsm/kg to have secretory diarrhea only if their stool weight exceeded 200 g/d. This was done because fecal fluid from normal people usually has an osmotic gap less than or equal to 50 mOsm/kg,[27,28] and if objective evidence of diarrhea was not required, most healthy people would meet the definition of secretory diarrhea.

Forty patients (25%) met criteria for classic secretory diarrhea without steatorrhea (see **Fig. 4**D) and other results of their stool analysis are summarized in **Table 3**. As stool weight increased, the sodium and chloride concentrations in fecal fluid increased and the potassium concentration decreased. Clinical disorders that typically cause classic secretory diarrhea without steatorrhea include microscopic colitis, stimulant laxatives (bisacodyl and senna), bacterial toxins, peptide hormones secreted by pancreatic endocrine tumors, epidemic chronic diarrhea (Brainerd diarrhea), self-limited secretory diarrhea, and congenital defects in electrolyte absorption. Most patients with classic secretory diarrhea caused by vasoactive intestinal polypeptide (VIP) secreting pancreatic endocrine tumors have stool weights exceeding 1000 g/d. There are many other diverse diseases that have been occasionally associated with secretory diarrhea without steatorrhea and the lists of these are available elsewhere.[4]

Recently, it was discovered that chronic secretory diarrhea can be caused by active potassium secretion by the colon, whereas colonic sodium absorption remains normal.[29–31] As a result, fecal fluid potassium concentration remains high as liquid stools develop, and fecal fluid sodium concentration remains low. Such patients tend to develop hypokalemia, probably caused by reduced food intake[32] and excess fecal loss of potassium. Stool analysis from one patient in this series showed this pattern (see **Table 3**). This form of secretory diarrhea has only been observed in patients with colonic ileus, and the authors consider the findings in this patient to establish that diagnosis. In **Fig. 4**B, this patient is denoted by the solid symbol.

Probable carbohydrate malabsorption without steatorrhea

Twenty-eight patients (18% of the total) met the criteria for probable carbohydrate malabsorption without steatorrhea. The results obtained in these 28 patients are individually depicted in **Table 4**. In general, the results in most of these 28 patients closely resemble the results that were obtained in a separate group of patients who developed diarrhea after ingesting lactose (see **Table 1**) wherein osmotic gaps were usually high and pH was usually greater than 5.5. Several of the findings are worthy of additional comment. First, stool weight was highly variable, from 121 to 4576 g/d. The patient whose stool weight was 4576 g/d had an osmotic gap of 206 mOsm/kg and a pH of 4.34 and this was similar to previous results on normal subjects who ingested large amounts of lactulose. Second, 26 of the patients had an osmotic gap greater than or equal to 75 mOsm/kg, 5 had a pH less than 5.5, and 3 patients met both criteria for carbohydrate malabsorption. Third, 2 of the patients with pH less than 5.5 had osmotic gaps of only 14 and 30 mOsm/kg, suggesting that virtually all of the unabsorbed carbohydrate had been metabolized to organic acids and that the diarrhea was mediated almost exclusively by sodium salts of organic acids. Fourth, when pH was greater than 5.5, it was often greater than 6.0, and was not approaching 5.5 in most cases. Fifth, the fecal fluid chloride was usually less in carbohydrate malabsorption than in secretory diarrhea.

The finding of probable carbohydrate malabsorption does not establish the specific cause of diarrhea but it indicates that the diarrhea is mediated at least partially by the osmotic effects of unabsorbed carbohydrates or organic acids derived from unab-sorbed carbohydrates. Nine of these 28 patients had stool weights greater than 500 g/d and the authors suspect that some of these had small bowel disease with secondary reduction in disaccharidase activity. Most patients had stool weights less than 500 g/d and these are more likely to have primary deficiencies of disaccharidases,

Table 3
Average results in patients with secretory diarrhea without steatorrhea

	Mean Stool Weight (g/d)	n	Mean [Na] (Range) (mEq/L)	Mean [K] (Range) (mEq/L)	Mean Ratio [Na]/[K] (Range)	Mean Osmotic Gap (Range) (mOsm/kg)	Mean [Cl] (Range) (mEq/L)	Mean Measured Osmolality (Range) (mOsm/kg)	Mean pH (Range)
Stool Weight Range (g/d)									
Classic									
200–500	302	15	69 (32–108)	65 (18–96)	1.41 (0.33–6.00)	22 (-16 to 6)	34 (15–91)	463 (370–690)	6.30 (5.68–6.68)
500–1000	673	13	89 (61–122)	46 (9–80)	3.35 (0.76–13.56)	20 (-6 to 48)	49 (10–97)	410 (335–478)	6.11 (5.22–6.84)
1000–2000	1283	9	94 (58–125)	41 (18–69)	2.86 (0.84–6.33)	23 (-6 to 48)	62 (42–82)	362 (286–460)	6.81 (5.91–8.53)
>2000	3605	2	103 (97–109)	32 (26–38)	3.30 (2.87–3.73)	20 (-4 to 44)	75 (65–85)	299 (291–306)	7.38 (6.71–8.05)
K-mediated	320	1	4	136	0.03	10	26	315	7.64

Table 4
Stool analysis results on 28 patients with carbohydrate malabsorption without steatorrhea

Patients	Stool Weight (g/d)	Consistency	Fecal Fat (g/d)	Concentration mEq/L				Osmotic Gap (mOsm/kg)	pH
				Na	K	Cl			
1	121	Formed, soft	1.1	37	64	19		88	6.26
2	127	Runny	0.4	68	37	72		80	8.36
3	133	Unformed, soft	3.6	31	75	26		78	6.48
4	166	Runny	1.7	59	30	33		112	6.95
5	169	Unformed, soft	1.9	46	55	17		88	5.89
6	175	Runny	1.4	63	39	50		86	6.22
7	178	Formed, soft	4.4	13	92	11		80	6.52
8	210	Runny	6.4	57	48	22		80	6.54
9	213	Unformed, soft	1.1	35	61	4		98	6.80
10	213	Mushy	3.6	30	52	18		126	6.42
11	221	Formed, soft	3.1	4	76	15		130	8.24
12	245	Unformed, soft	2.8	56	40	36		98	7.05
13	253	Mushy	3.0	47	19	27		158	7.34
14	264	Mushy	1.7	28	70	29		94	6.88
15	291	Unformed, soft	2.8	57	50	9		76	5.29
16	315	Unformed, soft	4.9	33	72	13		80	5.95
17	326	Runny	4.3	5	37	0		206	6.49
18	469	Runny	6.7	45	54	31		92	5.73
19	474	Runny	10.6	69	21	56		110	7.05
20	554	Mushy	6.5	27	62	15		112	6.41
21	593	Unformed, soft	2.3	32	52	16		122	7.34
22	694	Runny	1.2	61	77	10		14	5.22
23	707	Mushy	3.3	95	35	42		30	5.45
24	885	Runny	3.1	72	29	51		88	6.09
25	1070	Runny	3.7	70	30	19		90	7.01
26	1128	Watery	12.6	46	36	38		126	6.11
27	1296	Mushy	11.7	77	21	34		94	5.47
28	4576	Watery	16.0	31	11	10		206	4.34
	574 (121–4576)	Mean (range)	4.5 (0.4–16.0)	46 (4–95)	48 (11–92)	26 (0–72)		102 (14–206)	6.43 (4.34–8.36)

fructose malabsorption, or excess ingestion of fructose or sugar alcohols (such as sorbitol). Careful medical history can often trace the source of the offending carbohydrate to fruits, vegetables, or cereals in the diet, or to gums, soft drinks, nutritional supplements, health food products, or tube feedings. Carbohydrate malabsorption without steatorrhea might also be caused by iatrogenic or surreptitious ingestion of lactulose.

Steatorrhea with or without carbohydrate malabsorption

Forty patients had steatorrhea and stool weights greater than 200 g/d (see **Fig. 4D**) and 4 others had steatorrhea with stool weights less than 200 g/d (see **Table 2**, row 6). Steatorrhea was present in 8 patients with formed stools and in 4 of 15 patients with no objective evidence of diarrhea. The average fecal fat output in all 44 patients with steatorrhea was 28 g/d.

Fig. 5 shows the 44 patients with steatorrhea and plots the correlation between fecal fat output and stool weight. In general, fecal weight was higher in patients who had combined fat and carbohydrate malabsorption. The dotted line in **Fig. 5** shows the upper limit of normal for fecal fat output, which increases with increasing diarrheal stool weight (see "Definitions"). Fat output in some patients with steatorrhea was close to the dotted line, indicating mild steatorrhea, whereas the steatorrhea was severe in other patients.

In this study, 28% of patients with chronic idiopathic diarrhea had steatorrhea. In reviewing published work by other investigators, the authors found no previous data on the prevalence or severity of steatorrhea in a consecutive series of community-based patients presenting with chronic idiopathic diarrhea. The discovery of steatorrhea does not identify the cause of diarrhea but it would direct attention to small bowel and biliopancreatic diseases and away from surreptitious abuse of laxatives (except castor oil), microscopic colitis, and VIPoma syndrome.

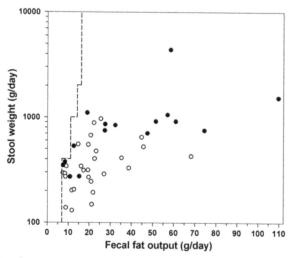

Fig. 5. Correlation between fecal fat output and stool weight in 44 patients with steatorrhea. Patients with steatorrhea without carbohydrate malabsorption are shown in open circles. Patients with steatorrhea and carbohydrate malabsorption are shown in solid circles. The dashed vertical line represents the output of fat in grams per day that is considered to be the upper limit of normal for varying degrees of diarrhea (see "Definitions").

Diarrhea induced by osmotic laxatives

Nine patients in this series had magnesium-induced diarrhea with stool weights that exceeded 200 g/d (see **Fig. 4E**). One additional patient had magnesium-induced diarrhea, but the stool weight was less than 200 g/d (see **Table 2**, row 4). In 2 of the 10 patients with magnesium-induced diarrhea, the magnesium concentration in fecal fluid exceeded 160 mEq/L (199 and 232 mEq/L), indicating that diarrhea was caused exclusively by excess magnesium intake. In 8 patients, the fecal magnesium concentrations were between 80 and 160 mEq/L (average 104, range 82–136 mEq/L), indicating that excess magnesium intake was responsible for a substantial fraction of the excess fecal water output but not for all of it. Further information from the patients and relatives would be required to determine if excess magnesium intake was inadvertent, iatrogenic, or intentional and surreptitious. Some of the sources of iatrogenic and inadvertent excess magnesium intake in patients with magnesium-induced diarrhea have been previously described.[24] As far as is known, magnesium-induced diarrhea does not result from malabsorption of magnesium ingested in normal foods because the quantity of magnesium in the diet is relatively small.

Osmotic diarrhea caused by PEG, such as that contained in lavage and laxative products like GoLytely and Miralax, is suspected when the osmotic gap is greater than 180 mOsm/kg and is confirmed by assay of fecal fluid for PEG.[17,18] As shown in **Fig. 4E**, one patient in this series had diarrhea caused by PEG (osmotic gap 228 mOsm/kg, PEG concentration 114 g/L, stool weight 491 g/d, and PEG output in stool 56 g/d).

Osmotic diarrhea caused by divalent anions (sulfate or phosphate) is suspected when the osmotic gap is negative, when the chloride concentration is low, and when the anion gap $([Na]+[K])-([Cl]+[HCO_3])$, where HCO_3 is bicarbonate and Cl is chloride, is greater than 110 mEq/L. The diagnosis is confirmed when fecal fluid contains high concentrations of these anions.[18,19] One patient in this series had osmotic diarrhea caused by excess intake of phosphate (presumably from a sodium phosphate–containing laxative) and that patient's results are shown in **Fig. 1**.

Unclassified patients, stool weight greater than 200 g/d

Thirteen of the 158 patients (8%) did not fit into any of the pathophysiological categories that the authors think have practical diagnostic value and they are designated as unclassified in **Fig. 4F**. Their osmotic gaps were between 52 and 70 mOsm/kg. Their daily stool weights varied from 205 to 1389 g/d.

Other Observations and Comments

Extremely high daily stool weights (>2000 g/d) occurred in 5 patients in this series. As shown in **Fig. 4**, 2 had secretory diarrhea without steatorrhea or carbohydrate malabsorption and they would be considered candidates for having an endocrine tumor releasing VIP or other secretory agonists. One patient had carbohydrate malabsorption without steatorrhea, one had severe steatorrhea (58.4 g/d) and carbohydrate malabsorption, and the final patient was ingesting an enormous amount of phosphate (see **Fig. 1**). Thus, extreme chronic diarrhea can have several different pathophysiological mechanisms.

Patients who surreptitiously ingest bisacodyl or senna to produce factitious diarrhea usually develop secretory diarrhea without steatorrhea. However, the authors do not send urine or stool from patients with these fecal fluid findings to a reference laboratory to test for bisacodyl or senna because a previous study showed that the only laboratory in the United States that offers such testing is highly unreliable, with false-positive results for bisacodyl and 100% false-negative results for senna.[11] In the United States, factitious diarrhea caused by senna and bisacodyl must be detected by other methods.[33] It should be noted that some patients take anthraquinone laxatives inadvertently via health food store products. A careful review of colon biopsies for melanosis coli can identify patients who have frequently ingested an anthraquinone during the previous year.

DISCUSSION AND SUMMARY

In the United States, patients are rarely admitted to the hospital for diagnostic studies alone. Therefore, if stool analysis is to have value as a diagnostic test, the method of stool collection would have to be feasible in both outpatients and inpatients. In general, the authors think that stool collections can be done as accurately at home as in the hospital. Obviously, this requires dedication to patient education.

It is hoped that the results presented here will allow gastroenterologists to judge for themselves whether or not stool analysis, as described herein, has practical value. Such judgment should be made with the best available knowledge of the relative charges for various procedures that are used in patients with chronic diarrhea and with best estimate of the frequency with which various procedures yield or point to a diagnosis. Medicare reimbursement to Baylor for comprehensive stool analysis is $99 (no other payments are made), whereas for colonoscopy with biopsies, the Medicare reimbursement to Baylor is $642 (and there are other payments to gastroenterologists, pathology laboratories, pathologists, and anesthesiologists). Thus, stool analysis is relatively inexpensive.

This retrospective analysis shows that stool analysis revealed helpful diagnostic information in 6 different ways. First, it identified a specific cause of diarrhea in 13 patients (8%): 12 were ingesting osmotic laxatives and 1 had potassium mediated secretory diarrhea, which is thought to occur only in patients with colonic ileus. Although an 8% specific diagnostic yield may seem small, the authors know of no other single procedure that has been shown to produce a higher specific yield in patients with chronic idiopathic diarrhea. Second, in 12 of 33 patients with stool weights less than 200 g/d, stool analysis revealed steatorrhea, probable carbohydrate malabsorption, or magnesium-induced diarrhea. Without comprehensive stool analysis, these 12 patients would probably have been labeled as having irritable bowel syndrome. Third, 28 of the patients in this series (18%) had evidence of carbohydrate malabsorption without steatorrhea. Diseases causing isolated carbohydrate malabsorption are unlikely to be detected by colonoscopy, mucosal biopsies, or imaging studies. However, once suspected by stool analysis, such causes can often be identified by focused medical history, exclusion diets and hydrogen breath tests. Fourth, steatorrhea was found in 44 patients in this series (28%), pointing to diseases that interfere with fat absorption or digestion. In some instances it would be useful to know that a patient has steatorrhea before upper endoscopy is done to obtain a duodenal biopsy. For example, if celiac serology was negative, in addition to duodenal biopsy, the endoscopist could obtain jejunal fluid for anaerobic culture and parasites and duodenal fluid after secretin injection to evaluate exocrine pancreatic function.[34] Fifth, 21 female patients in this series had secretory diarrhea without steatorrhea, suggesting the possibility of factitious diarrhea caused by bisacodyl or senna. By detailed and focused review of social and past medical history, and by speaking to relatives and the patients' previous physicians, a fraction of these 21 patients would be identified as high risk for surreptitious ingestion of these laxatives. Sixth, 11 patients had secretory diarrhea without steatorrhea and stool weights greater than 1000 g/d, placing them at risk for a pancreatic endocrine tumor; 2 patients in this group had stool weights greater than 3000 g/d, placing them at high risk for this syndrome.

This retrospective analysis also revealed or confirmed limitations of stool analysis. First, like endoscopy and imaging studies, stool analysis cannot specifically diagnose most of the causes of diarrhea listed at the end of the first paragraph of the introduction. Therefore, in most patients with chronic idiopathic diarrhea, a specific cause would not be forthcoming even if comprehensive stool analysis is used. Moreover, in cases that are not diagnosed by stool analysis, there is no proof that results of stool analysis would lead to the discovery of a specific cause that would otherwise have been missed. Such proof would require a randomized prospective study, with the order of procedures performed according to protocol, and a predetermined definition of what constitutes a diagnosis. Second, there is no doubt that stool analysis, as performed in the authors' laboratory, is not ideal and is limited in scope. A detailed record of dietary fat intake would allow steatorrhea to be defined by the percentage of dietary fat that is excreted in stool,[35] as well as by fecal fat output. Knowledge of carbohydrate intake would help in the interpretation of carbohydrate malabsorption. Additional analytical procedures (total carbohydrate, organic acids, reducing sugars) would provide a better definition of carbohydrate malabsorption, and an accurate test for bisacodyl- and senna-induced diarrhea would increase the specific diagnostic yield of stool analysis. Offering supplemental stool analysis to evaluate transit time of a water-soluble marker, adjusted for the severity of diarrhea, would provide insight into the role of hypermotility in chronic diarrhea,[36] which is not assessed by any of the diagnostic tests or procedures that are now used.

Balancing the useful diagnostic information that was obtained, the limitations that exist, and the cost of various diagnostic procedures, the authors think that stool analysis, as used here, has substantial practical diagnostic value in patients with chronic diarrhea. If it were used early in the diagnostic evaluation, the authors think it would reduce the cost of making a diagnosis and that it would reduce the overutilization of invasive, potentially dangerous procedures. Placing stool analysis under the auspices of gastroenterology rather than laboratory services may be a prerequisite for its successful deployment as a diagnostic procedure. The authors agree with gastroenterologists who think stool analysis should be improved rather than discarded.[37]

ACKNOWLEDGMENTS

The authors are grateful to Beiqi Xue, Jack Porter, and Lawrence Schiller for their careful review of this article and their excellent editorial suggestions. Michael Emmett gave valuable advice on the interpretation of electrolyte and pH changes in carbohydrate malabsorption. Kenneth Fine read and edited the article on multiple occasions, made many constructive comments, and contributed to all aspects of interpreting the results and writing the final article.

REFERENCES

1. Young VB, Schmidt TM. Antibiotic-associated diarrhea accompanied by large-scale alterations in the composition of the fecal microbiota. J Clin Microbiol 2004;42(3):1203–6.
2. Read NW, Krejs GJ, Read MG, et al. Chronic diarrhea of unknown origin. Gastroenterology 1980;78(2):264–71.
3. Fordtran JS, Santa Ana CA, Morawski SG, et al. Pathophysiology of chronic diarrhoea: insights derived from intestinal perfusion studies in 31 patients. Clin Gastroenterol 1986;15(3):477–90.

4. Fine KD, Krejs GJ, Fordtran JS. Diarrhea. In: Sleisenger MH, Fordtran JS, editors. Gastrointestinal disease: pathophysiology, diagnosis, management. 5th edition. Philadelphia: Saunders; 1993. p. 1043–69.

5. Amaratunge C, Sellin JH. Evaluation of patients with diarrhea and timing of referral. In: Guandalini S, Vaziri H, editors. Diarrhea: diagnostic and therapeutic advances. New York: Springer; 2011. p. 431–42.

6. Fedorak RN, Rubinoff MJ. Basic investigation of a patient with diarrhea. In: Field M, editor. Diarrheal diseases. New York: Elsevier; 1991. p. 191–218.

7. Fine KD, Schiller LR. AGA technical review on the evaluation and management of chronic diarrhea. Gastroenterology 1999;116(6):1464–86.

8. Hill PG. Faecal fat: time to give it up. Ann Clin Biochem 2001;38:164–7.

9. Thomas PD, Forbes A, Green J, et al. Guidelines for the investigation of chronic diarrhea, 2nd edition. Gut 2003;52:v1–15.

10. Holbrook I. The British Society of Gastroenterology guidelines for the investigation of chronic diarrhea, 2nd edition. Ann Clin Biochem 2005;42:170–4.

11. Shelton JH, Santa Ana CA, Thompson DR, et al. Factitious diarrhea induced by stimulant laxatives: accuracy of diagnosis by a clinical reference laboratory using thin layer chromatography. Clin Chem 2007;53(1):85–90.

12. van de Kamer JH, TEN Bokkel Huinink H, Weyers HA. Rapid method for the determination of fat in feces. J Biol Chem 1949;177:347–55.

13. Smith JS, Ediss I, Mullinger MA, et al. Fecal chymotrypsin and trypsin determinations. Can Med Assoc J 1971;104(8):691–7.

14. Fine KD, Fordtran JS. The effect of diarrhea on fecal fat excretion. Gastroenterology 1992;102:1936–9.

15. Comfort MW, Wollaeger EE, Taylor AB, et al. Nontropical sprue: observations on absorption and metabolism. Gastroenterology 1953;23:155–78.

16. Wollaeger EE, Comfort MW, Osterberg AE. Total solids, fat and nitrogen in the feces: III. A study of normal persons taking a test diet containing a moderate amount of fat; comparison with results obtained with normal persons taking a test diet containing a large amount of fat. Gastroenterology 1947;9:272–83.

17. Hammer HF, Santa Ana CA, Schiller LR, et al. Studies of osmotic diarrhea induced in normal subjects by ingestion of polyethylene glycol and lactulose. J Clin Invest 1989;84:1056–62.

18. Eherer AJ, Fordtran JS. Fecal osmotic gap and pH in experimental diarrhea of various causes. Gastroenterology 1992;103:545–51.

19. Fine KD, Ogunji F, Florio R, et al. Investigation and diagnosis of diarrhea caused by sodium phosphate. Dig Dis Sci 1998;43(12):2708–14.

20. Hammer HF, Fine KD, Santa Ana CA, et al. Carbohydrate malabsorption: its measurement and its contribution to diarrhea. J Clin Invest 1990;86:1936–44.

21. Perman JA, Modler S, Olson AC. Role of pH in production of hydrogen from carbohydrates by colonic bacterial flora. J Clin Invest 1981;67:643–50.

22. Ameen VZ, Powell GK. A simple spectrophotometric method for quantitative fecal carbohydrate measurement. Clin Chim Acta 1985;152:3–9.

23. Caspary WF. Diarrhoea associated with carbohydrate malabsorption. Clin Gastroenterol 1986;15(3):631–55.

24. Fine KD, Santa Ana CA, Fordtran JS. Diagnosis of magnesium-induced diarrhea. N Engl J Med 1991;324:1012–7.

25. Eherer AJ, Santa Ana CA, Porter J, et al. Effect of psyllium, calcium polycarbophil, and wheat bran on secretory diarrhea induced by phenolphthalein. Gastroenterology 1993;104:1007–12.

26. Wenzl HH, Fine KD, Schiller LR, et al. Determinants of decreased fecal consistency in patients with diarrhea. Gastroenterology 1995;108:1729–38.

27. Wrong O, Metcalfe-Gibson A, Morrison RB, et al. In vivo dialysis of faeces as a method of stool analysis. I. Technique and results in normal subjects. Clin Sci 1965;28:357–75.

28. Bjork JT, Soergel KH, Wood CM. The composition of "free" stool water. Gastroenterology 1975;70:864.

29. van Dinter TG, Fuerst FC, Richardson CT, et al. Stimulated active potassium secretion in a patient with colonic pseudo-obstruction: a new mechanism of secretory diarrhea. Gastroenterology 2005;129:1268–73.

30. Blondon H, Béchade D, Desramé J, et al. Secretory diarrhoea with high fecal potassium concentrations: a new mechanism of diarrhoea associated with colonic pseudo-obstruction? Report of five patients. Gastroenterol Clin Biol 2008;32(4):401–4.

31. Simon M, Duong JP, Mallet V, et al. Over-expression of colonic K+ channels associated with severe potassium secretory diarrhea after haemorrhagic shock. Nephrol Dial Transplant 2008;23:3350–2.

32. Agarwal R, Afzalpurkar R, Fordtran JS. Pathophysiology of potassium absorption and secretion by the human intestine. Gastroenterology 1994;107:548–71.

33. Savino AC, Fordtran JS. Factitious disease: clinical lessons from case studies at Baylor University Medical Center. Proc (Bayl Univ Med Cent) 2006;19:195–208.

34. Stevens T, Conwell DL, Zuccaro G, et al. Electrolyte composition of endoscopically collected duodenal drainage fluid after synthetic porcine secretin stimulation in healthy subjects. Gastrointest Endosc 2004;60:351–5.

35. Odstrcil EA, Martinez JG, Santa Ana CA, et al. The contribution of malabsorption to the reduction in net energy absorption after long-limb Roux-en-Y gastric bypass. Am J Clin Nutr 2010;92:704–13.

36. Guirl MJ, Högenauer C, Santa Ana CA, et al. Rapid intestinal transit as a primary cause of severe chronic diarrhea in patients with amyloidosis. Am J Gastroenterol 2003;98:2219–25.

37. Lust M, Nandurkar S, Gibson PR. Measurement of faecal fat excretion: an evaluation of attitudes and practices of Australian gastroenterologists. Intern Med J 2006;36:77–85.

Colorectal Normal Histology and Histopathologic Findings in Patients with Chronic Diarrhea

Cord Langner, MD

KEYWORDS

- Microscopic colitis • Mast cell colitis • Inflammatory bowel disease
- Ulcerative colitis • Crohn's disease • Diverticular disease–associated colitis (DAC)

KEY POINTS

- Close communication between gastroenterologists and pathologists is necessary for accurate classification of patients with chronic diarrhea because there is considerable histologic overlap among different disease entities.
- Endoscopy with random mucosal biopsy is the only means of verifying the diagnosis of microscopic colitis, and its importance has been widely recognized.
- Mast cell (mastocytic) colitis has recently emerged as another condition associated with chronic diarrhea, but its significance still has to be defined.
- Preserved mucosal architecture is the histologic hallmark of microscopic colitis and distinguishes the disease from inflammatory bowel disease, particularly ulcerative colitis in remission.

INTRODUCTION

Diarrhea is defined in terms of stool frequency, consistency, volume, or weight. Acute diarrhea is usually caused by infections or toxic agents. In contrast, chronic diarrhea usually has noninfectious causes. Although there is no general consensus on the duration of symptoms that differentiate acute from chronic diarrhea, most clinicians will agree that symptoms persisting for longer than 4 weeks suggest a noninfectious cause and merit further investigation. Six to 8 weeks, however, may provide a clearer distinction.[1] According to the guidelines published by the British Society of Gastroenterology, chronic diarrhea is defined as the abnormal passage of 3 or more loose or liquid stools per day for more than 4 weeks or a daily stool weight greater than 200 g/d.[2]

The author has nothing to disclose.
Institute of Pathology, Medical University of Graz, Auenbruggerplatz 25, Graz 8036, Austria
E-mail address: cord.langner@medunigraz.at

Gastroenterol Clin N Am 41 (2012) 561–580
http://dx.doi.org/10.1016/j.gtc.2012.06.005
0889-8553/12/$ – see front matter © 2012 Elsevier Inc. All rights reserved.

The prevalence of chronic diarrhea varies depending on definition and the studied population and has been reported to be 4% to 5% in the general population and 7% to 14% in an elderly population.[3,4] Routine workup often includes endoscopic evaluation of the small and large bowel, and histological assessment of mucosal biopsies is an integral part of this procedure. In a study that has examined the prevalence of colonic pathologic conditions in patients with non–HIV-related chronic diarrhea, 15% of patients had histologic abnormalities. The most common diagnoses were microscopic (lymphocytic and collagenous) colitis, Crohn's disease, and ulcerative colitis.[5] Routine ileoscopy may enhance the diagnostic yield, and it has been suggested that in patients with chronic diarrhea, colonoscopy and ileoscopy with biopsy may lead to a definitive diagnosis in approximately 15% to 20% of cases.[2] Although the examination of a biopsy specimen without clinical information can avoid cognitive bias, the full benefit of the pathologist's experience and opinion can only be obtained if appropriate clinical information is available.[6]

According to the American Gastroenterological Association's technical review on the evaluation and management of chronic diarrhea,[1] the disorders that can be diagnosed by endoscopic mucosal inspection mainly include Crohn's disease and ulcerative colitis, but melanosis coli, ulceration, and large colorectal polyps and tumors may also be identified as underlying causes. Diseases with mucosae that seem normal on endoscopic inspection but are associated with histologic abnormalities include microscopic colitis, amyloidosis, and some rare infections.

This review starts with a description of the normal anatomy because awareness of the range of normal, noninflamed, colorectal histology may help to avoid clinically useless terms, such as mild inflammatory changes or mild nonspecific colitis/proctitis. In its main section, the review focuses on the different forms of microscopic colitis, including mast cell (mastocytic) enterocolitis, and on the histopathology of inflammatory bowel disease (IBD), including various aspects of differential diagnosis.

NORMAL HISTOLOGY

The colorectal mucosa is flat and has no villi, as opposed to normal small bowel mucosa. Sections cut perpendicular to the surface show the crypts as straight tubes in parallel alignment that extend from immediately above the muscularis mucosae to the mucosal surface. The crypts are more or less closely packed and evenly distributed (>6 per millimeter).[6] The distances between the individual crypts and their internal diameters are fairly stable, yet some variation and slight alterations in crypt configuration can be present in healthy individuals, particularly in the region of lymphoid follicles and innominate groves. Under normal conditions, the branching of crypts is rarely observed (<1 per millimeter). In a well-oriented section, crypt shortening (atrophy) is generally absent. Of note, mild uniform crypt shortening can reflect tangential cutting and is of no importance if the biopsy specimen is otherwise normal.[6,7]

The luminal surface of the mucosa is covered by a single-cell layer of columnar epithelium composed of absorptive and goblet cells, resting on a thin, regular collagen table. Lymphocytes (CD3+/CD8+ T cells) may occasionally be present between surface cells (intraepithelial lymphocytes [IEL]), their number not exceeding 5 per 100 epithelial cells.[6] The cell population lining the crypts is more complex. In addition to mature absorptive and goblet cells, neuroendocrine and Paneth cells are found, the latter only in the caecum and ascending colon. At the base of the crypts, immature precursor (stem) cells reside within the so-called stem cell niche.[8] These pluripotent cells are capable of unlimited self-renewal and divide asymmetrically with one daughter cell residing in the niche and the other daughter cell migrating upward along the crypt axis. These latter cells are named transient amplifying cells. They represent the main proliferation compartment within the crypt and ultimately differentiate into the 4 mature cell types described earlier. In the luminal part of the crypt, cells have lost the ability to divide, but they become more functionally mature until they eventually exfoliate from the surface. This journey along the crypt axis normally takes between 72 and 192 hours, leading to renewal of the colonic surface epithelium every 3 to 8 days.

Inflammatory cells are normally present in varying numbers within the lamina propria and are responsible for the local immunologically mediated host defense. The cells are diffusely distributed, with most cells localized in the superficial third of the mucosa (superficial vs basal third 2:1). In addition, up to 2 lymphoid aggregates or follicles in a 2-mm biopsy specimen may be regarded as normal. Thus, these cells *do not* represent chronic inflammation (**Fig. 1**).

Under normal conditions, plasma cells (B cells) are the predominant round cell, and T lymphocytes and macrophages represent other common inhabitants of the lamina propria. Myeloid cells that are normally present include eosinophils and mast cells. Their number is highly variable, but they are relatively rare; eosinophils account for approximately 3.5% and mast cells account for approximately 2% of the cells within

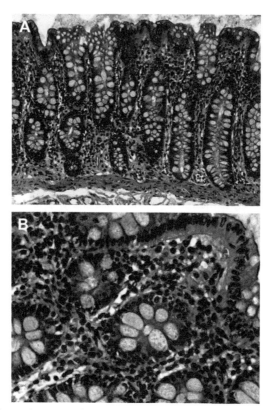

Fig. 1. Normal colorectal mucosa of a 64-year-old man, distal resection margin of a right hemicolectomy specimen for colorectal carcinoma. Note the inflammatory cells are normally present in varying numbers within the lamina propria, predominantly in the superficial third of the mucosa (hematoxylin-eosin, original magnification ×100) (*A*). On high power, the infiltrate mainly consists of mononuclear cells, particularly lymphocytes and plasma cells (hematoxylin-eosin, original magnification ×200) (*B*). These cells do not represent chronic inflammation.

the lamina propria.[9] The detection of mast cells requires special staining. Of note, mast cell numbers that are assessed by immunohistochemistry (antibodies directed against tryptase, KIT/CD117) are higher than those detected by toluidine blue staining because the latter method only stains the minority of activated cells (ie, degranulated cells), which may predominate in areas of inflammation.[9] Neutrophils should not be present normally in either the surface or the crypt epithelium.

The cellular composition of the lamina propria varies between different anatomic segments of the large bowel. The density of mucosal lymphocytes is significantly higher in the right colon than in the left colon and particularly the rectum.[10,11] Likewise, the absolute and relative number of mast cells within the lamina propria is lowest in the rectosigmoid, whereas the number of eosinophils does not change significantly from segment to segment.[9,10]

Within the lamina propria, fibroblasts are found randomly distributed throughout the lamina propria. Their number is highest in the most superficial portion of the lamina propria adjacent to the basement membrane of the surface epithelium as well as encompassing the crypts (pericryptal myofibroblasts). There is considerable crosstalk between these latter cells and the cells within the stem cell niche, which is essential for mucosal integrity and differentiation.[12,13] Immediately below the basement membrane complex of superficial epithelial cells, a collagen layer is found that is no thicker than 3 to 5 μm.[6,14] Of note, tangential cutting of biopsy specimens may cause apparent expansion of the basement membrane. Together with the eosinophilic subnuclear zone of surface epithelial cells, this may give a false impression of a thickened subepithelial collagen layer.[6,15]

MICROSCOPIC COLITIS
Collagenous and Lymphocytic Colitis

Microscopic colitis is a common cause of chronic or recurrent watery (nonbloody) diarrhea. The term was initially coined in 1980 to describe patients with chronic watery diarrhea and minor histologic changes with no other evident causes despite extensive workup.[16] Currently, microscopic colitis is used as an umbrella term that includes 2 major conditions without endoscopic or radiologic lesions but with histologic abnormalities that are traditionally termed *collagenous colitis* and *lymphocytic colitis*.[14,17,18]

Collagenous colitis was first described in 1976 in a woman with chronic diarrhea, normal barium enema and sigmoidoscopy, and findings of a thickened subepithelial collagen band and an increased IEL count on histology.[19] The term lymphocytic colitis was introduced in 1989 in a similar clinical and histologic context without the finding of a thickened subepithelial collagen band.[20] It is likely that the two conditions are part of a spectrum because the clinical features are similar and there is substantial overlap in histologic findings. In a recent investigation, histologic findings suggested coexistence with the other type of microscopic colitis in 48% of patients with collagenous colitis and in 24% of patients with lymphocytic colitis, respectively.[21]

In a large epidemiologic study from Sweden, microscopic colitis accounted for approximately 10% of all patients investigated for chronic (nonbloody) diarrhea and for almost 20% of those older than 70 years.[22] The number of patients diagnosed with lymphocytic colitis is similar to that of collagenous colitis.[18] The disease occurs predominantly in older adults, with the diagnosis most commonly made in the sixth to seventh decade (average age at diagnosis is 53–69 years). However, a wide age range has been reported, including pediatric cases.[14,18,23] Women are more commonly affected than men, with a female-to-male ratio ranging from 3:1 to 9:1 for collagenous colitis and 1:1 to 6:1 for lymphocytic colitis, respectively.[18] The incidence has increased over time to levels comparable with other forms of IBD. The reason for this increase is not clear, but growing awareness of the disease may be partially responsible.[14] One study showed that microscopic colitis is diagnosed less commonly in small nonacademic centers.[24]

The pathogenesis of microscopic colitis is largely unknown. Most cases are idiopathic, but an abnormal immunologic reaction to a luminal antigen (eg, infectious agents and drugs, such as proton pump inhibitors and nonsteroidal antiinflammatory drugs [NSAIDs]), possibly in a genetically predisposed individual, seems to play a major role.[25,26] Notably, 20% to 60% of patients with lymphocytic colitis and 17% to 40% of patients with collagenous colitis suffer from autoimmune diseases, such as rheumatoid arthritis, collagen vascular diseases, or thyroid disorders. There is also a strong association with celiac disease,[27] which is detected in 6% to 27% of patients with lymphocytic colitis and 8% to 17% of patients with collagenous colitis, respectively. In a recent study evaluating the incidence of microscopic colitis in a large database of patients with celiac disease, microscopic colitis was found in 44 of 1009 patients (4.3%), which corresponds to a 70-fold increased risk compared with that in the general population.[28]

The excessive collagen deposition in collagenous colitis has been related to alterations in subepithelial myofibroblast function, possibly leading to matrix or collagen overproduction.[29] However, impaired degradation of extracellular matrix proteins (ie, impaired fibrolysis) may also play a major role.[30]

Although by definition, in microscopic colitis the mucosa of the large intestine should be normal on endoscopic inspection, subtle changes, such as mild edema and erythema as well as an abnormal vascular pattern, may occasionally be seen.[14,23] If colonic ulcers are present, these are likely to be caused by NSAIDs.[31]

The key histologic feature of microscopic colitis is an increased number of surface IEL with little to no disruption of the mucosal architecture (**Fig. 2**A).[14] On sections stained with hematoxylin and eosin (H&E), IEL are characterized by mostly round, compact nuclei with a dense chromatin pattern, slightly irregular nuclear outline, and perinuclear halo. Most investigators refer to a cutoff of 20 or more IEL per 100 surface epithelial cells, but some also refer to 15 or more IEL (median 30, range 10–66).[17] The terminal ileum may be affected in both lymphocytic and collagenous colitis. One study analyzing ileal biopsies from patients with lymphocytic and collagenous colitis (none of them had celiac disease) proved the presence of 5 or more IEL per 100 surface epithelial cells to be highly specific for microscopic colitis.[32] Compared with healthy individuals, there is increased mononuclear inflammation within the lamina propria with even distribution (ie, loss of the normally decreasing inflammatory cell density gradient toward the muscularis mucosae) (see **Fig. 2**B). Neutrophils may also be present, and active cryptitis with occasional crypt abscess formation has been reported to occur in 30% to 38% of patients, although acute inflammation should not predominate within the inflammatory infiltrate.[33]

In patients with collagenous colitis, a thickened collagen layer is seen underneath the surface epithelium, which is most evident between crypts (see **Fig. 2**C). Most investigators agree that the thickness of the collagen layer should exceed 10 μm (often 15–30 μm, up to 70 μm) on well-oriented biopsies (ie, biopsies cut perpendicular to the mucosal surface). Diarrhea is commonly noted when the collagen layer exceeds 15 μm.[17] Care should be taken to avoid the misinterpretation of a tangentially cut basement membrane (see earlier discussion). In selected cases, additional stains, such as trichrome staining or tenascin immunohistochemistry, may be helpful.[29] The collagen entraps capillaries and inflammatory cells, leading to nuclear abnormalities of enclosed lymphocytes (twisted lymphocytes).

Secondary changes to the surface epithelium are common and are usually more pronounced in collagenous than in lymphocytic colitis. They include flattening or

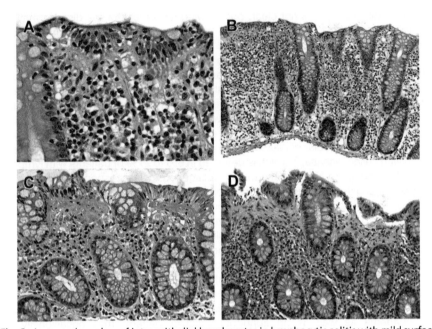

Fig. 2. Increased number of intraepithelial lymphocytes in lymphocytic colitis with mild surface epithelial damage (hematoxylin-eosin, original magnification ×200) (*A*). Increased predominantly mononuclear inflammation within the lamina propria (hematoxylin-eosin, original magnification ×100) (*B*). Thickening of the subepithelial collagen layer in collagenous colitis, most evident in between crypts (hematoxylin-eosin, original magnification ×150) (*C*). Note characteristic detachment of surface epithelial cells from subepithelial collagen and increased cellularity within the lamina propria (hematoxylin-eosin, original magnification ×125) (*D*).

degeneration (cytoplasmic vacuoles, pyknotic nuclei) of columnar cells, or both, and mucin depletion. In collagenous colitis, the detachment of surface epithelial cells from subepithelial collagen represents a common histologic feature (see **Fig. 2**D). Occasionally, focal IBD-like inflammatory changes and Paneth cell metaplasia in the right colon (44% in collagenous colitis, 14% in lymphocytic colitis) may be observed.[33] Crypt distortion, shortening (atrophy), or branching, however, are not features of microscopic colitis.[33,34] In fact, the overall absence of crypt architectural irregularities in lymphocytic and collagenous colitis is the major difference between microscopic colitis and IBD.[17] **Box 1** summarizes the key morphologic features of lymphocytic and collagenous colitis.

The reliability of using flexible sigmoidoscopy in making the diagnosis is of some controversy.[14] Nonuniform distribution of the subepithelial collagen band has been reported in collagenous colitis with less thickening in the rectosigmoid.[35] Likewise, IEL counts were found to be increased in the right compared with the left colon in lymphocytic colitis.[36] As a consequence, earlier studies mostly recommended the use of colonoscopy in the workup of patients with chronic diarrhea in order not to miss affected individuals. However, in a large systematic investigation of 809 patients evaluated for chronic diarrhea who had no endoscopically visible abnormalities on colonoscopy, 80 (10%) were found to have microscopic colitis, all of whom had evidence of disease in the left colon.[5] In another recent study, 95% of patients with collagenous colitis and 98% of patients with lymphocytic colitis had diagnostic

---

Box 1
Microscopic colitis: key histologic features of lymphocytic and collagenous colitis

Lymphocytic colitis

- Increased number of surface intraepithelial lymphocytes ($\geq$20 per 100 epithelial cells)
- Surface epithelial damage (flattening, mucin depletion)
- Increased (and homogeneously distributed) mononuclear inflammation in the lamina propria (plasma cells > lymphocytes)
- Thickening (<10 μm) of subepithelial collagen layer possible
- Focal IBD-like changes (cryptitis, Paneth cell metaplasia) possible

Collagenous colitis

- Diffusely distributed and thickened subepithelial collagen layer greater than or equal to 10 μm (not all samples may be involved)
- Surface epithelial damage (flattening, detachment)
- Increased (and homogeneously distributed) mononuclear inflammation in the lamina propria (plasma cells > lymphocytes)
- Increased number of surface intraepithelial lymphocytes possible
- Focal IBD-like changes (cryptitis, Paneth cell metaplasia) possible

---

histopathology in both the right and the left colon, and normal histology in biopsies obtained from the left colon had a high negative predictive value for microscopic colitis.[21] Biopsy material obtained only from the rectum, however, is known to have low sensitivity with respect to the diagnosis of microscopic colitis.[11,37,38]

Thus, the advantages of flexible sigmoidoscopy over total colonoscopy must be weighed against the marginally increased diagnostic yield of colonoscopy regarding microscopic colitis. Colonoscopy may be reserved for those patients in whom results of distal biopsies obtained on sigmoidoscopy were normal or inconclusive. In these patients, a full colonoscopic examination with sampling of both the transverse and the ascending colon should be completed.[39,40] However, this suggestion is limited to patients thought to have microscopic colitis and should not be extended to the evaluation of patients with diarrhea in general because it does not take into account proximal colonic lesions (eg, caused by Crohn's disease), which may only be accessible by colonoscopy.

Variants of Microscopic Colitis

The spectrum of morphologic changes associated with chronic watery (nonbloody) diarrhea seems to be broader than originally thought. In 30% of patients, there are only minor histologic abnormalities, such as increased cellular density (plasma cells and lymphocytes) within the lamina propria, whereas IEL counts are not significantly elevated (between 5 and 20 per 100 surface epithelial cells) and the subepithelial collagen bands measure only between 5 and 10 μm in thickness.

Because these patients do not fulfill the criteria for classic lymphocytic colitis or collagenous colitis, they are usually not treated. Follow-up endoscopic biopsies, however, may render changes diagnostic for microscopic colitis; according to a recent study, as much as 30% of cases of microscopic colitis are diagnosed only on repeated endoscopy.[21]

Some investigators have offered the term *microscopic colitis not otherwise specified* (NOS) for these cases,[11,41] whereas others refer to these cases with incomplete findings of microscopic colitis as *atypical microscopic colitis*,[42] *incomplete microscopic colitis,*[21] or *paucicellular lymphocytic colitis.*[43,44] It has been suggested to sign out these cases in a more descriptive way as *epithelial lymphocytosis (not diagnostic for lymphocytic colitis)*, and other conditions should be considered, such as a late phase of infectious colitis.[17,42] The identification and reporting of these borderline cases could be the pathologist's contribution to reduce the risk of missing patients with a treatable cause of diarrhea.[21]

It currently remains unsolved whether patients with classic lymphocytic and collagenous colitis and patients with incomplete histologic findings should be regarded as one clinical entity.[21] A recent immunohistologic study evaluating the expression of CD25+ regulatory T cells and FOXP3 in mucosal biopsies has shown discordant profiles in classic lymphocytic colitis and paucicellular lymphocytic colitis. This finding suggests different pathogenetic mechanisms, thereby arguing against paucicellular lymphocytic colitis as a minor form of classic lymphocytic colitis.[44]

The term *cryptal lymphocytic coloproctitis* has been introduced to describe patients with chronic watery (nonbloody) diarrhea and significant intraepithelial lymphocytosis within the crypt epithelium, yet not within the surface epithelium.[45] Patients with this peculiar histologic pattern are rare, and the significance of the diagnosis is largely unknown. Microscopic colitis with giant cells refers to the presence of multinucleated giant cells within the lamina propria in otherwise classic lymphocytic or collagenous colitis.[46,47] These giant cells are of histiocytic origin and seem to form through histiocyte fusion. Their presence does not seem to confer any clinical significance and may be regarded as a histologic curiosity.[48]

Other reported rare variants or presumed subtypes of microscopic colitis, such as pseudomembranous collagenous colitis[49] and microscopic colitis with granulomatous inflammation,[50] have been described. It is currently unclear whether these are specific entities. An overview is given in **Fig. 3**. Furthermore, several other conditions are characterized by diarrhea without endoscopically visible lesions but with abnormal histology. Examples are intestinal spirochetosis, postinfectious irritable bowel syndrome, and IBD in remission; for a review, see Geboes.[17]

MAST CELL (MASTOCYTIC) ENTEROCOLITIS

Mast cells represent a normal constituent of the lamina propria. They contain granules rich in histamine and are well known for their role in allergy and anaphylaxis. Although their exact function is still only partially understood, mast cells are increasingly recognized as playing an important protective role and being intimately involved in the defense against different pathogens. In the gastrointestinal tract, mast cells are involved in several disorders, including irritable bowel syndrome and IBD.[14]

The gastrointestinal tract may rarely be involved in cases of systemic mastocytosis, an uncommon condition characterized by abnormal proliferation (D816 V *KIT* mutation) of mast cells in one or more organs. Most cases are confined to the skin, but 10% involve extracutaneous sites, most commonly bone, liver, spleen, gastrointestinal tract, and lymph nodes.[51,52] All parts of the gastrointestinal tract may be affected. In the colon, the gross/endoscopic appearance may be similar to that in IBD, showing mucosal nodularity and erosions. Histologically, the lamina propria is diffusely infiltrated with mast cells arranged in sheets or aggregates. Some mucosal architectural distortion is present in most cases. Of note, mast cells may display several phenotypes on routinely H&E-stained slides, some of which may be mistaken for eosinophils or histiocytes.[52]

The terms *mast cell colitis* or *mastocytic enterocolitis* have been used primarily in 2 publications to characterize patients with chronic diarrhea, normal mucosa on

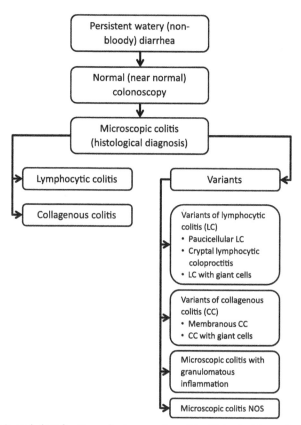

Fig. 3. Diagnosis and classification of microscopic colitis. (*Adapted from* Chang F, Deere H, Vu C. Atypical forms of microscopic colitis: morphologic features and review of the literature. Adv Anat Pathol 2005;12:203–11.)

endoscopic inspection, and increased mast cell count in mucosal biopsies.[53,54] The author has recently published the case of a 49-year-old man with chronic diarrhea and marked mast cell infiltration of the lamina propria. Treatment with histamine receptor antagonists led to rapid and persistent amelioration of clinical symptoms.[55]

As pointed out previously, the number of mucosal mast cells is highly variable, and the cutoff of 20 or more mast cells per high-power field recommended by Jakate and colleagues[53] to define abnormal mast cell infiltration is arbitrary and still needs external validation. In addition, it is currently not clear whether mast cell (mastocytic) enterocolitis is a specific diagnosis or whether increased mast cell numbers are caused by their widespread residence within the gastrointestinal tract as potential mediators of inflammation.[14] Nevertheless, the detection of increased mast cell numbers in patients with chronic, intractable diarrhea may offer a new therapeutic perspective.

Because mast cells cannot definitively be identified on routinely H&E-stained slides, additional stains are necessary for the quantification of mast cell density. Immunostaining using antibodies directed against mast cell tryptase or KIT renders mast cell numbers that are higher than those obtained with toluidine blue staining (see earlier discussion). Close cooperation between gastroenterologists and pathologists is essential to identify patients who might benefit from this procedure.

INFLAMMATORY BOWEL DISEASE
Histologic Features of Crohn's Disease and Ulcerative Colitis

The analysis of multiple biopsies allows a correct diagnosis of IBD in 66% to 75% of newly diagnosed patients. Providing additional endoscopic and clinical data to the pathologist increases the diagnostic accuracy, allowing a final diagnosis in more than 90% of cases.[56,57]

According to Jenkins and colleagues,[6] the histologic features useful for a diagnosis of IBD may be grouped into 4 categories: mucosal architecture, lamina propria cellularity, neutrophil polymorph infiltration, and epithelial abnormality. In the following, these features will be referred to in detail.

- Various abnormalities in crypt architecture are a hallmark feature of IBD. They are particularly pronounced in ulcerative colitis (57%–100% of cases) but may also occur in Crohn's disease (27%–71% of cases).[6] Among these abnormalities, crypt distortion implies the presence of nonparallel crypts of varying diameter. Crypt branching reflects regenerative changes; the presence of more than 2 branched crypts within a well-oriented biopsy with at least 2 mm length of muscularis mucosae may be regarded as abnormal.[6] Crypt shortening (atrophy) reflects the presence of an increased, usually variable, distance between the bases of the crypts and the muscularis mucosae. Severe crypt architectural abnormalities may lead to surface irregularities (eg, pseudovillous change). Another architectural feature of IBD is reduced crypt density, so that adjacent crypts are separated by lamina propria equivalent to 1 or more crypt diameter.[6]
- In IBD, the cellularity of the lamina propria is commonly increased (88%–93% of cases). There is a characteristic change in the ratio between superficial and deep levels that results in diffuse transmucosal infiltration of mononuclear cells, preferably plasma cells. The latter are typically identified between the bases of the crypts and the muscularis mucosae (basal plasmacytosis). A discontinuous chronic inflammation is seen more often in Crohn's disease (26% of cases) than in ulcerative colitis (10% of cases), in which a discontinuous pattern has been related to therapy effects (compare with later discussion). Non-necrotic epithelioid cell granulomas are present in approximately 30% to 50% of cases with Crohn's disease. Of note, they may be found in all layers of the bowel wall and can be identified in mucosal biopsies only in approximately 20% of cases.[58] Granulomas may also be found in ulcerative colitis (up to 5% of cases) where they are almost invariably seen around ruptured crypts (cryptolytic granulomas), representing a foreign-body–type histiocytic response to extravasated mucin.[59,60]
- The presence of acute inflammation (ie, infiltration of lamina propria, surface or crypt epithelium [cryptitis, crypt abscess formation]) by neutrophils indicates disease activity, together with features of acute surface epithelial damage (erosions, ulcerations).
- Epithelial abnormalities consistent with subacute or chronic epithelial damage mainly include surface epithelial damage (flattening, vacuolation, focal cell loss), mucin depletion (reduction in the number of goblet cells), and metaplastic change. Mucin depletion is more frequent in ulcerative colitis (35%–69% of cases) than in Crohn's disease (5%–57% of cases).[6] Metaplasia occurs as Paneth cell metaplasia in the left colon, mainly in ulcerative colitis, or as pyloric gland metaplasia in the terminal ileum of patients with Crohn's disease.

Depending on the phase of the disease, mucosal biopsies from patients with ulcerative colitis or Crohn's disease may show evidence of active inflammation or chronic injury.[61] Microscopic features that favor a diagnosis of ulcerative colitis are severe, diffuse (continuous) crypt atrophy or distortion, decreased crypt density, and a frankly irregular mucosal surface. In addition, a marked, diffuse, transmucosal increase of predominantly mononuclear inflammatory cells (with basal plasmacytosis) and the detection of Paneth cells in biopsies obtained distal to the hepatic flexure are highly suggestive of the disease. Tissue fragments both within the same biopsy and within separately submitted specimens tend to show the same degree of inflammation (**Fig. 4**).[62]

By contrast, features that favor a diagnosis of Crohn's disease are discontinuous crypt architectural abnormalities (eg, focal crypt atrophy or distortion) and discontinuous inflammation (eg, focal cryptitis). Focal or patchy inflammation may be observed in biopsies submitted from different parts of the bowel or may be present within tissue fragments of the same biopsy, not rarely within a single biopsy specimen.[62] Mucosal defects typically occur in the form of fissuring ulcers and aphthous erosions. Epithelioid cell granulomas not related to crypt damage or rupture are not necessary for diagnosis but, if present, they may render an additional diagnostic clue (**Fig. 5**). In surgical specimens, the presence of transmural lymphoid aggregates (specificity 90%, positive predictive value 62%), fibromuscular obliteration and nerve fiber hyperplasia in the submucosa are common.[63] **Box 2** summarizes the key histologic features of ulcerative colitis and Crohn's disease.

Approximately 50% of patients with Crohn's disease have colonic involvement, and nearly 20% develop colitis without involvement of the esophagus, stomach, or small intestine.[58] According to Warren,[64] there are 3 basic patterns of colorectal involvement: Crohn's disease isolated to the rectum (with perianal fissures and fistulae),

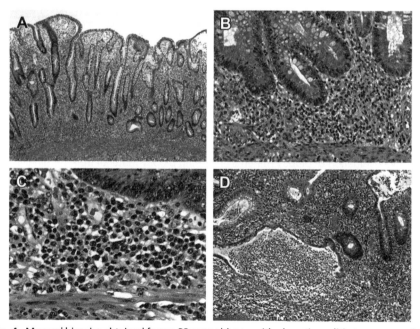

Fig. 4. Mucosal biopsies obtained from a 32-year-old man with ulcerative colitis. Low-power view showing diffuse (continuous) crypt atrophy and distortion (hematoxylin-eosin, original magnification ×100) (*A*). Note Paneth cell metaplasia at the bottom of the crypts (hematoxylin-eosin, original magnification ×150) (*B*). There is a marked, diffuse, transmucosal increase of predominantly mononuclear inflammatory cells with basal plasmacytosis (hematoxylin-eosin, original magnification ×300) (*C*). Disease activity is demonstrated by the presence of neutrophils in the lamina propria and by crypt abscess formation (hematoxylin-eosin, original magnification ×100) (*D*).

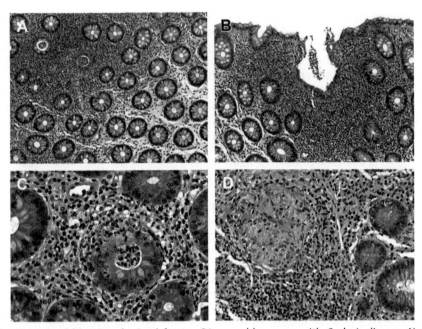

Fig. 5. Mucosal biopsies obtained from a 21-year-old woman with Crohn's disease. Note preserved crypt architecture and discontinuous mucosal inflammation (hematoxylin-eosin, original magnification ×100) (*A*). Characteristic aphthous erosion (hematoxylin-eosin, original magnification ×100) (*B*) and active cryptitis (hematoxylin-eosin, original magnification ×300) (*C*). An epithelioid cell granuloma not related to crypt damage or rupture is seen in the lamina propria next to the muscularis mucosae (hematoxylin-eosin, original magnification ×150) (*D*).

stricturing large bowel Crohn's disease, and diffuse Crohn's colitis. Discriminating diffuse Crohn's colitis from ulcerative colitis represents a major challenge for pathologists. In surgical specimens, the diagnosis relies heavily on the presence of granulomas and transmural lymphoid aggregates. If only biopsy material is available, an extensive evaluation of biopsy material (including biopsy material from terminal ileum and upper gastrointestinal tract) for the presence of hardcore features of Crohn's disease, combined with correlation with the clinical and endoscopic features of the patient, is mandatory.[58,61,65]

The terminal ileum is involved in 40% of patients with Crohn's disease.[63] The involvement of the distal few centimeters of the ileum may occasionally be observed in ulcerative colitis. In a study by Haskell and colleagues,[66] inflammatory changes in the ileum were identified in 34 of 200 (17%) patients with ulcerative colitis and all but 2 patients (94%) had pancolitis. Changes were generally mild in nature (villous atrophy, increased inflammation, scattered crypt abscesses). The pathogenesis of these findings is largely unclear, but reflux of colonic contents (backwash ileitis) has been discussed as a potential cause.[61,65]

In the upper gastrointestinal tract, focal active gastritis that is more common in the antrum than in the gastric body and focal active duodenitis have a high predictive value for Crohn's disease.[64,67] According to recent literature data, however, upper gastrointestinal tract involvement may also occur in ulcerative colitis, particularly in children.[68–71] The significance of this finding is currently unclear. Opportunistic infection caused by immunosuppressive therapy has to be ruled out.[72]

> **Box 2**
> **IBD: key histologic features of ulcerative colitis and Crohn's disease**
>
> *Ulcerative colitis*
>
> • Diffuse (continuous) mucosal disease that begins in the rectum and spreads variably to the proximal colon (worse distally)
>
> • Severe diffuse mucosal architectural abnormalities (crypt atrophy and distortion, decreased crypt density)
>
> • Severe diffuse transmucosal increase in lamina propria inflammatory cells (predominantly mononuclear cells)
>
> • Rare fissures, superficial in fulminant colitis
>
> • Epithelial abnormalities, such as surface epithelial damage (flattening) and mucin depletion and Paneth cell metaplasia
>
> • Rare epithelioid cell granulomas, related to ruptured crypts
>
> *Crohn's disease*
>
> • Segmental (discontinuous) transmural disease (skip lesions with fissures, fistulae) with variable rectal involvement and variable disease severity (worse proximally)
>
> • Focal (discontinuous) crypt architectural abnormalities (focal crypt atrophy and distortion)
>
> • Focal (discontinuous) inflammation (focal mononuclear expansion of the lamina propria, focal cryptitis)
>
> • Aphthous erosions/ulcers and deep fissures, any location
>
> • Epithelioid cell granulomas (not crypt related) in approximately 20% of mucosal biopsies
>
> • Transmural lymphoid aggregates and fibromuscular obliteration and nerve fiber hyperplasia in the submucosa on surgical specimens

Problems in Diagnosis and Differential Diagnosis

Ulcerative colitis and Crohn's disease show overlapping morphologic features, and a precise diagnosis may be difficult, if not impossible, in 10% to 15% of cases.[57] In fact, there is no single pathognomonic histologic feature, and the diagnosis typically rests on a combination of clinical, laboratory, endoscopic, and histologic observations, with ulcerative colitis showing more severe architectural and inflammatory abnormalities than Crohn's disease.[63,65,73]

In specimens from patients operated on for severe (fulminant) colitis, making a definitive diagnosis may be particularly challenging. For these cases, the terms *colitis of uncertain type* or *indeterminate colitis* have been introduced.[73] If the diagnosis cannot reliably be established on biopsy specimens, the term *IBD unclassified* should be applied. Because all of these terms do not reflect a distinct entity, there are no specific histologic features and no diagnostic criteria.[58] In fact, these diagnoses are usually considered to be provisional descriptive terms or temporary diagnoses, and follow-up biopsies help to establish a more precise diagnosis. In up to 80% of patients, the true nature of the patients' underlying IBD becomes apparent within a few years, and most cases represent ulcerative colitis on long-term follow-up.[58,73–75]

The differential diagnosis between ulcerative colitis and Crohn's disease may also be challenging when patients are undergoing therapy. Both local and systemic treatments have a major impact on histology, causing diagnostic histologic features and the features indicating disease activity to vary with time and treatment.[76] Thus, mucosal healing in ulcerative colitis may cause discontinuous inflammation.[61,77] Moreover, rectal sparing that is normally seen in ulcerative colitis in up to 30% of pediatric patients, but not in adults, may occur in adults following topical or systemic therapy.[78,79] A recent systematic analysis of patients with IBD who underwent procto-colectomy showed that rectal sparing following therapy is in fact only relative and not absolute.[80] In that study, most patients showed patchy, minor inflammatory changes that had been missed in earlier random biopsies obtained from endoscopically normal mucosa. Thus, for accurate typing of IBD, the pathologist needs to know whether the patient is under treatment.[57] A diagnostic algorithm taking treatment effects into consideration is presented in **Fig. 6**.

Apart from the treatment effects, discontinuous inflammation of the colon in ulcerative colitis may be seen in patients with left-sided disease as focal inflammation of the cecum (cecal patch) or ascending colon or as appendiceal involvement.[61,81–83] Most patients with ulcerative colitis show a sharp demarcation between affected and unaffected parts of their large bowel, but some patients may show a more gradual transition.[81] The transition zone may seem somewhat patchy, and analysis of biopsy material obtained from this area may give the false impression of discontinuous inflammation.[76]

In early onset disease (2–6 weeks after the first symptoms), the histologic features that are most useful in separating IBD from other inflammatory conditions, such as crypt architectural abnormalities and basal plasmacytosis, may not have been established fully. Early reaction to pathogens is characterized by the accumulation of neutrophils, whereas an increase in mononuclear cells, particularly lymphocytes and plasma cells, occurs at a later phase of the disease, as do architectural abnormalities, which result from more widespread and repetitive epithelial injury.[57] Thus, in one study, plasmacytosis increased from 38% in biopsies obtained 1 to 15 days following the onset of symptoms to 89% in biopsies obtained after 121 to 300 days. Architectural abnormalities started 16 to 30 days after the onset of symptoms and increased from 0% to 78%.[84] Likewise, metaplastic changes are observed only in long-standing disease.

Conditions that may mimic IBD mainly include prolonged (persistent) infection and diverticular disease-associated colitis; other differential diagnoses to be considered are microscopic colitis with features of IBD, radiation injury, NSAID-induced colitis, diversion colitis, and chronic recurrent ischemic colitis.[58,65] Prolonged infection may lead to mild abnormalities in mucosal architecture. However, as in acute self-limiting colitis, cryptitis and crypt abscess formation is more common in the superficial third of the mucosa (as opposed to ulcerative colitis), and features of chronicity, such as basal plasmacytosis, are almost invariably lacking.[61]

The presence of a superimposed secondary disease, often related to the use of immunosuppressive drugs, may mask the true nature of the underlying IBD.[58] For example, infection by cytomegalovirus may simulate a flare of the patients' underlying IBD, which is typically refractory to (intensified) immunosuppressive therapy.[61] Infection with *Clostridium difficile* causing histologic features of pseudomembranous colitis represents another example.[58]

Diverticular disease-associated colitis (DAC), also known as segmental colitis associated with diverticulosis (SCAD), develops in 1.5% to 3.8% of patients with diverticulosis.[62] Almost invariably, there is segmental involvement of the sigmoid (and distal descending) colon, whereas the more proximal parts of the colon and the rectum are not involved. Endoscopy typically reveals mucosal erythema, friability, and ulceration, which is similar to changes in ulcerative colitis. On histology, chronic colitis with crypt architectural abnormalities, mixed inflammatory infiltrate, cryptitis, and crypt abscess formation as well as basal plasmacytosis and occasional Paneth cell metaplasia can be observed in the interdiverticular luminal mucosa. Even transmural lymphoid aggregates and epithelioid cell granulomas may be seen.[85] Thus, DAC/SCAD and IBD may be

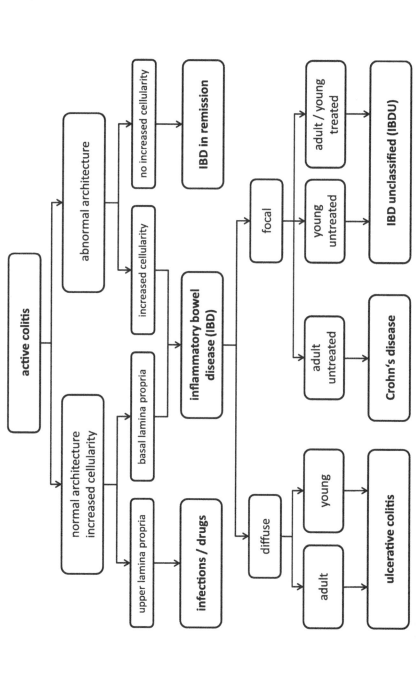

Fig. 6. Histopathologic algorithm for the diagnosis of colitis. (*Adapted from* Geboes K, van Eyken P. Inflammatory bowel disease unclassified and indeterminate colitis: the role of the pathologist. J Clin Pathol 2009;62:201–5.)

virtually indistinguishable on morphologic analysis, and the diagnosis of DAC/SCAD should always be considered when entertaining a diagnosis of IBD in patients with disease limited to the sigmoid (and lower descending) colon with rectal sparing.[58,62,86] The pathogenesis of DAC/SCAD remains elusive. Goldstein and colleagues[85] speculated that the inflammatory changes may represent an idiosyncratic mucosal response to bacterial stasis and inflammation within diverticula or to relative ischemia.

SUMMARY

Close communication between gastroenterologists and pathologists is necessary for accurate classification of patients with chronic diarrhea because there is considerable histologic overlap among different disease entities.

Collagenous and lymphocytic colitis are fairly common causes of chronic, watery (nonbloody) diarrhea without endoscopically visible lesions but with histologic abnormalities and are, therefore, summarized as microscopic colitis. Currently, endoscopy with random mucosal biopsy is the only means of verifying the diagnosis, and its importance has been widely recognized. Several variants of microscopic colitis have been described, but it is unclear whether these represent specific entities.

Recently, mast cell (mastocytic) colitis has emerged as another condition associated with chronic diarrhea; its significance, however, still has to be defined. Of note, mast cells cannot be identified unequivocally on routinely H&E-stained slides. Their assessment requires special stains, preferably immunohistochemistry. Therefore, gastroenterologists need to inform pathologists if mast cell colitis is clinically suspected in order not to miss affected individuals.

Preserved mucosal architecture is the histologic hallmark of microscopic colitis and distinguishes the disease from IBD, particularly ulcerative colitis in remission. In addition to architectural abnormalities, the diagnosis of IBD rests on characteristic inflammatory changes. Their severity and distribution in a biopsy series are important for differential diagnosis together with other features, such as mucin depletion, granuloma formation, metaplastic change, and ileal involvement. Certain histologic features characteristic for Crohn's disease may also occur in ulcerative colitis and vice versa. Differential diagnosis mainly includes prolonged infection and diverticular disease–associated colitis.

REFERENCES

1. Fine KD, Schiller LR. AGA technical review on the evaluation and management of chronic diarrhea. Gastroenterology 1999;116:1464–86.
2. Thomas PD, Forbes A, Green J, et al. Guidelines for the investigation of chronic diarrhoea, 2nd edition. Gut 2003;52(Suppl 5):v1–15.
3. Talley NJ, O'Keefe EA, Zinsmeister AR, et al. Prevalence of gastrointestinal symptoms in the elderly: a population-based study. Gastroenterology 1992;102: 895–901.
4. Talley NJ, Weaver AL, Zinsmeister AR, et al. Onset and disappearance of gastrointestinal symptoms and functional gastrointestinal disorders. Am J Epidemiol 1992;136:165–77.
5. Fine KD, Seidel RH, Do K. The prevalence, anatomic distribution, and diagnosis of colonic causes of chronic diarrhea. Gastrointest Endosc 2000;51:318–26.
6. Jenkins D, Balsitis M, Gallivan S, et al. Guidelines for the initial biopsy diagnosis of suspected chronic idiopathic inflammatory bowel disease. The British Society of Gastroenterology Initiative. J Clin Pathol 1997;50:93–105.
7. Levine DS, Haggitt RC. Normal histology of the colon. Am J Surg Pathol 1989;13: 966–84.

8. Zeki SS, Graham TA, Wright NA. Stem cells and their implications for colorectal cancer. Nat Rev Gastroenterol Hepatol 2011;8:90–100.

9. Bischoff SC, Wedemeyer J, Herrmann A, et al. Quantitative assessment of intestinal eosinophils and mast cells in inflammatory bowel disease. Histopathology 1996;28:1–13.

10. Chadwick VS, Chen W, Shu D, et al. Activation of the mucosal immune system in irritable bowel syndrome. Gastroenterology 2002;122:1778–83.

11. Warren BF, Edwards CM, Travis SP. 'Microscopic colitis': classification and terminology. Histopathology 2002;40:374–6.

12. Brabletz S, Schmalhofer O, Brabletz T. Gastrointestinal stem cells in development and cancer. J Pathol 2009;217:307–17.

13. Kosinski C, Stange DE, Xu C, et al. Indian hedgehog regulates intestinal stem cell fate through epithelial-mesenchymal interactions during development. Gastroenterology 2010;139:893–903.

14. Yen EF, Pardi DS. Review article: microscopic colitis–lymphocytic, collagenous and 'mast cell' colitis. Aliment Pharmacol Ther 2011;34:21–32.

15. Nyhlin N, Bohr J, Eriksson S, et al. Systematic review: microscopic colitis. Aliment Pharmacol Ther 2006;23:1525–34.

16. Read NW, Krejs GJ, Read MG, et al. Chronic diarrhea of unknown origin. Gastroenterology 1980;78:264–71.

17. Geboes K. Lymphocytic, collagenous and other microscopic colitides: pathology and the relationship with idiopathic inflammatory bowel diseases. Gastroenterol Clin Biol 2008;32:689–94.

18. Pardi DS, Kelly CP. Microscopic colitis. Gastroenterology 2011;140:1155–65.

19. Lindström CG. 'Collagenous colitis' with watery diarrhoea–a new entity? Pathol Eur 1976;11:87–9.

20. Lazenby AJ, Yardley JH, Giardiello FM, et al. 'Lymphocytic ("microscopic") colitis: a comparative histopathologic study with particular reference to collagenous colitis. Hum Pathol 1989;20:18–28.

21. Bjørnbak C, Engel PJ, Nielsen PL, et al. Microscopic colitis: clinical findings, topography and persistence of histopathological subgroups. Aliment Pharmacol Ther 2011;34:1225–34.

22. Olesen M, Eriksson S, Bohr J, et al. Microscopic colitis: a common diarrhoeal disease. An epidemiological study in Orebro, Sweden, 1993-1998. Gut 2004;53:346–50.

23. Temmerman F, Baert F. Collagenous and lymphocytic colitis: systematic review and update of the literature. Dig Dis 2009;27(Suppl 1):137–45.

24. Harewood GC, Olson JS, Mattek NC, et al. Colonic biopsy practice for evaluation of diarrhea in patients with normal endoscopic findings: results from a national endoscopic database. Gastrointest Endosc 2005;61:371–5.

25. Fernández-Bañares F, Esteve M, Espinós JC, et al. Drug consumption and the risk of microscopic colitis. Am J Gastroenterol 2007;102:324–30.

26. Keszthelyi D, Jansen SV, Schouten GA, et al. Proton pump inhibitor use is associated with an increased risk for microscopic colitis: a case-control study. Aliment Pharmacol Ther 2010;32:1124–8.

27. Stewart M, Andrews CN, Urbanski S, et al. The association of coeliac disease and microscopic colitis: a large population-based study. Aliment Pharmacol Ther 2011;33:1340–9.

28. Green PH, Yang J, Cheng J, et al. An association between microscopic colitis and celiac disease. Clin Gastroenterol Hepatol 2009;7:1210–6.

29. Salas A, Fernández-Bañares F, Casalots J, et al. Subepithelial myofibroblasts and tenascin expression in microscopic colitis. Histopathology 2003;43:48–54.

30. Günther U, Schuppan D, Bauer M, et al. Fibrogenesis and fibrolysis in collagenous colitis. Patterns of procollagen types I and IV, matrix-metalloproteinase-1 and -13, and TIMP-1 gene expression. Am J Pathol 1999;155:493–503.

31. Kakar S, Pardi DS, Burgart LJ. Colonic ulcers accompanying collagenous colitis: implication of nonsteroidal anti-inflammatory drugs. Am J Gastroenterol 2003;98: 1834–7.

32. Sapp H, Ithamukkala S, Brien TP, et al. The terminal ileum is affected in patients with lymphocytic or collagenous colitis. Am J Surg Pathol 2001;26:1484–92.

33. Ayata G, Ithamukkala S, Sapp H, et al. Prevalence and significance of inflammatory bowel disease-like morphologic features in collagenous and lymphocytic colitis. Am J Surg Pathol 2002;26:1414–23.

34. Nielsen OH, Vainer B, Rask-Madsen J. Non-IBD and noninfectious colitis. Nat Clin Pract Gastroenterol Hepatol 2008;5:28–39.

35. Tanaka M, Mazzoleni G, Riddell RH. Distribution of collagenous colitis: utility of flexible sigmoidoscopy. Gut 1992;33:65–70.

36. Thijs WJ, van Baarlen J, Kleibeuker JH, et al. Microscopic colitis: prevalence and distribution throughout the colon in patients with chronic diarrhoea. Neth J Med 2005;63:137–40.

37. Carpenter HA, Tremaine WJ, Batts KP, et al. Sequential histologic evaluations in collagenous colitis. Correlations with disease behavior and sampling strategy. Dig Dis Sci 1992;37:1903–9.

38. Agnarsdottir M, Gunnlaugsson O, Orvar KB, et al. Collagenous and lymphocytic colitis in Iceland. Dig Dis Sci 2002;47:1122–8.

39. Datta I, Brar SS, Andrews CN, et al. Microscopic colitis: a review for the surgical endoscopist. Can J Surg 2009;52:E167–72.

40. Yantiss RK, Odze RD. Optimal approach to obtaining mucosal biopsies for assessment of inflammatory disorders of the gastrointestinal tract. Am J Gastroenterol 2009;104:774–83.

41. Fraser AG, Warren BF, Chandrapala R, et al. Microscopic colitis: a clinical and pathological review. Scand J Gastroenterol 2002;37:1241–5.

42. Chang F, Deere H, Vu C. Atypical forms of microscopic colitis: morphological features and review of the literature. Adv Anat Pathol 2005;12:203–11.

43. Goldstein NS, Bhanot P. Paucicellular and asymptomatic lymphocytic colitis: expanding the clinicopathologic spectrum of lymphocytic colitis. Am J Clin Pathol 2004;122:405–11.

44. Fernández-Bañares F, Casalots J, Salas A, et al. Paucicellular lymphocytic colitis: is it a minor form of lymphocytic colitis? A clinical pathological and immunological study. Am J Gastroenterol 2009;104:1189–98.

45. Rubio CA, Lindholm J. Cryptal lymphocytic coloproctitis: a new phenotype of lymphocytic colitis? J Clin Pathol 2002;55:138–40.

46. Libbrecht L, Croes R, Ectors N, et al. Microscopic colitis with giant cells. Histopathology 2002;40:335–8.

47. Sandmeier D, Bouzourene H. Microscopic colitis with giant cells: a rare new histopathologic subtype? Int J Surg Pathol 2004;12:45–8.

48. Brown IS, Lambie DL. Microscopic colitis with giant cells: a clinico-pathological review of 11 cases and comparison with microscopic colitis without giant cells. Pathology 2008;40:671–5.

49. Yuan S, Reyes V, Bronner MP. Pseudomembranous collagenous colitis. Am J Surg Pathol 2003;27:1375–9.

50. Saurine TJ, Brewer JM, Eckstein RP.Saurine TJ, et al. Microscopic colitis with granulomatous inflammation. Histopathology 2004;45:82–6.

51. Hahn HP, Hornick JL. Immunoreactivity for CD25 in gastrointestinal mucosal mast cells is specific for systemic mastocytosis. Am J Surg Pathol 2007;31: 1669–76.
52. Kirsch R, Geboes K, Shepherd NA, et al. Systemic mastocytosis involving the gastrointestinal tract: clinicopathologic and molecular study of five cases. Mod Pathol 2008;21:1508–16.
53. Jakate S, Demeo M, John R, et al. Mastocytic enterocolitis: increased mucosal mast cells in chronic intractable diarrhea. Arch Pathol Lab Med 2006;130: 362–7.
54. Ogilvie-McDaniel C, Blaiss M, Osborn FD, et al. Mastocytic enterocolitis: a newly described mast cell entity. Ann Allergy Asthma Immunol 2008;101:645–6.
55. Thonhofer R, Siegel C, Trummer M, et al. Mastocytic enterocolitis as a rare cause of chronic diarrhea in a patient with rheumatoid arthritis. Wien Klin Wochenschr 2011;123:297–8.
56. Bentley E, Jenkins D, Campbell F, et al. How could pathologists improve the initial diagnosis of colitis? Evidence from an international workshop. J Clin Pathol 2002; 55:955–60.
57. Geboes K, van Eyken P. Inflammatory bowel disease unclassified and indeterminate colitis: the role of the pathologist. J Clin Pathol 2009;62:201–5.
58. Yantiss RK, Odze RD. Diagnostic difficulties in inflammatory bowel disease pathology. Histopathology 2006;48:116–32.
59. Lee FD, Maguire C, Obeidat W, et al. Importance of cryptolytic lesions and pericryptal granulomas in inflammatory bowel disease. J Clin Pathol 1997;50:148–52.
60. Warren BF, Shepherd NA, Price AB, et al. Importance of cryptolytic lesions and pericryptal granulomas in inflammatory bowel disease. J Clin Pathol 1997;50:880–1.
61. Yantiss RK, Odze RD. Pitfalls in the interpretation of nonneoplastic mucosal biopsies in inflammatory bowel disease. Am J Gastroenterol 2007;102: 890–904.
62. Patel S, Voltaggio L. A practical approach to colitis. Diagn Histopathol 2011;17: 376–85.
63. Geboes K. What histologic features best differentiate Crohn's disease from ulcerative colitis? Inflamm Bowel Dis 2008;14:S168–9.
64. Warren BF. Classic pathology of ulcerative and Crohn's colitis. J Clin Gastroenterol 2004;38:S33–5.
65. Odze RD. Diagnostic problems and advances in inflammatory bowel disease. Mod Pathol 2003;16:347–58.
66. Haskell H, Andrews CW Jr, Reddy SI, et al. Pathological features and clinical significance of "backwash" ileitis in ulcerative colitis. Am J Surg Pathol 2005; 29:1472–81.
67. Oberhuber G, Püspök A, Oesterreicher C, et al. Focally enhanced gastritis: a frequent type of gastritis in patients with Crohn's disease. Gastroenterology 1997;112:698–706.
68. Sharif F, McDermott M, Dillon M, et al. Focally enhanced gastritis in children with Crohn's disease and ulcerative colitis. Am J Gastroenterol 2002;97:1415–20.
69. Hori K, Ikeuchi H, Nakano H, et al. Gastroduodenitis associated with ulcerative colitis. J Gastroenterol 2008;43:193–201.
70. Danelius M, Ost A, Lapidus AB. Inflammatory bowel disease-related lesions in the duodenal and gastric mucosa. Scand J Gastroenterol 2009;44:441–5.
71. Lin J, McKenna BJ, Appelman HD. Morphologic findings in upper gastrointestinal biopsies of patients with ulcerative colitis: a controlled study. Am J Surg Pathol 2010;34:1672–7.

72. Harbaum L, Siebert F, Langner C. Opportunistic streptococcal gastritis in a patient with ulcerative colitis mimicking gastric involvement by inflammatory bowel disease. Inflamm Bowel Dis 2010;16:2008–9.

73. Geboes K, De Hertogh G. Indeterminate colitis. Inflamm Bowel Dis 2003;9: 324–31.

74. Meucci G, Bortoli A, Riccioli FA, et al. Frequency and clinical evolution of indeterminate colitis: a retrospective multi-centre study in northern Italy. GSMII (Gruppo di Studio per le Malattie Infiammatorie Intestinali). Eur J Gastroenterol Hepatol 1999;11:909–13.

75. Odze RD. Pathology of indeterminate colitis. J Clin Gastroenterol 2004;38: S36–40.

76. Guindi M, Riddell RH. Indeterminate colitis. J Clin Pathol 2004;57:1233–44.

77. Kim B, Barnett JL, Kleer CG, et al. Endoscopic and histological patchiness in treated ulcerative colitis. Am J Gastroenterol 1999;94:3259–62.

78. Glickman JN, Bousvaros A, Farraye FA, et al. Pediatric patients with untreated ulcerative colitis may present initially with unusual morphologic findings. Am J Surg Pathol 2004;28:190–7.

79. Glickman JN, Odze RD. Does rectal sparing ever occur in ulcerative colitis? Inflamm Bowel Dis 2008;14:S166–7.

80. Joo M, Odze RD. Rectal sparing and skip lesions in ulcerative colitis: a comparative study of endoscopic and histologic findings in patients who underwent proctocolectomy. Am J Surg Pathol 2010;34:689–96.

81. D'Haens G, Geboes K, Peeters M, et al. Patchy cecal inflammation associated with distal ulcerative colitis: a prospective endoscopic study. Am J Gastroenterol 1997;92:1275–9.

82. Matsumoto T, Nakamura S, Shimizu M, et al. Significance of appendiceal involvement in patients with ulcerative colitis. Gastrointest Endosc 2002;55:180–5.

83. Mutinga ML, Odze RD, Wang HH, et al. The clinical significance of right-sided colonic inflammation in patients with left-sided chronic ulcerative colitis. Inflamm Bowel Dis 2004;10:215–9.

84. Schumacher G, Kollberg B, Sandstedt B. A prospective study of first attacks of inflammatory bowel disease and infectious colitis. Histologic course during the 1st year after presentation. Scand J Gastroenterol 1994;29:318–32.

85. Goldstein NS, Leon-Armin C, Mani A. Crohn's colitis-like changes in sigmoid diverticulitis specimens is usually an idiosyncratic inflammatory response to the diverticulosis rather than Crohn's colitis. Am J Surg Pathol 2000;24:668–75.

86. Peppercorn MA. The overlap of inflammatory bowel disease and diverticular disease. J Clin Gastroenterol 2004;38:S8–10.

Bacterial Flora as a Cause or Treatment of Chronic Diarrhea

Franco Scaldaferri, MD, Marco Pizzoferrato, MD, Silvia Pecere, MD,
Fabrizio Forte, MD, Antonio Gasbarrini, MD*

KEYWORDS

• Gut microbiota • Chronic diarrhea • Intestinal homeostasis • Probiotics • Antibiotics

KEY POINTS

• Chronic diarrhea is related to a disregulation of intestinal homeostasis and gut microflora composition.
• Gut microbiota is involved in maintaining mucosal integrity, in immune system modulation, toxin metabolism, and trophic functions. Its alteration is found in many conditions like irritable bowel syndrome (IBS), small intestinal bacterial overgrowth (SIBO) and inflammatory bowel disease (IBD).
• There are several techniques for studying gut microbiota: indirect methods like breath tests or direct methods including cultures, microbial gene microarray analysis, fluorescent in situ hybridization, and ribosomal RNA analysis.
• Prebiotics and probiotics are able to modulate intestinal microflora, regulate mucosal immunity, and preserve epithelial integrity in many entheropathies.
• The correct use of antibiotics can modulate gut microbiota and reduce symptoms of many gastrointestinal conditions like IBS, IBD, and SIBO.

INTRODUCTION

The digestive tract is constantly interacting with the external environment, being the major immunologic organ of the body. It is responsible for immune tolerance as well as for immune activation in case of infections. Most of these functions are made possible by the continuous crosstalk between gastrointestinal mucosa and microorganisms contained in the intestine, commonly called gut microbiota. The gut microbiota, the whole intestinal flora of the gastrointestinal tract, is a complex microbiological system that is attracting increasing interest from the scientific community. It is estimated that the total number of bacteria in the human body is 10 to 100 trillion, at least 10 times more than the total number of somatic and germ cells of the human body,[1] with bacterial genes in a ratio of 100:1 with human genes.[2]

Financial disclosures: None.
Division of Internal Medicine and Gastroenterology, Policlinico A. Gemelli Hospital - Catholic University of Rome, Igo Gemelli 8, Rome 00168, Italy
* Corresponding author.
E-mail address: agasbarrini@rm.unicatt.it

Gastroenterol Clin N Am 41 (2012) 581–602
http://dx.doi.org/10.1016/j.gtc.2012.06.002
0889-8553/12/$ – see front matter © 2012 Elsevier Inc. All rights reserved.

To date, studies of gut microbiota have been limited because of technical issues in the identification and study of microbial components.[3] The number of species present in human intestine is between 500 and 800, of which 80% cannot be cultured in the laboratory with available techniques,[4] but new methods are now available, at least for research purposes, and include denaturing gradient gel electrophoresis (DGGE) analysis and microarray, and these techniques are already changing the understanding about the physiology of the digestive system.[5]

MUCOSAL BARRIER, GUT MICROBIOTA, AND INTESTINAL HEALTH

Gut microbiota can be considered an organ in the human body, and, because of its continuous and constant crosstalk with intestinal mucosa, it supports several physiologic processes including the intestinal barrier effect, immune system modulation (inducing tolerance and/or activation), metabolic and trophic functions through production of butyric acid or other products, drug and toxin metabolism, and behavior conditioning.[6–8] These functions are possible because of its direct or indirect interaction with components of the intestinal mucosa. Direct interaction occurs with enterocytes, dendritic cells and intraepithelial immune cells. Indirect interaction occurs for immune cells and nonimmune cells or the noncell population of the intestinal mucosa. Immune cells within the lamina propria are mononuclear cells, lymphocytes, polymorphonuclear cells, plasma cells, dendritic cells, and macrophages. Immune cells are organized, particularly in the small intestine, in microstructures, called Peyer patches, and in lymphoid tissue associated with gastrointestinal mucosa. Nonimmune cells, whose role in intestinal homeostasis is also important, are mesenchymal cells, endothelial cells, fibroblasts, and muscular and nervous cells.[9–12]

Under physiologic conditions, there is a continuous recirculation of immune cells from peripheral blood to lymph nodes: this balance is defined as physiologic inflammation caused by antigens of the normal intestinal flora and diet.[9]

The recognition of antigens depends on specific or nonspecific mechanisms. Nonspecific mechanisms are responsible, for instance, for the recognition of lipopolysaccharides or peptidoglycans, and are shared by diverse cellular subtypes responsible for innate immunity. Toll-like receptors (TLRs) and NOD-like receptors (NLRs), the most important innate immunity pathways, are the major armamentarium for both immune and nonimmune cells to sense gut microbiota. In contrast, specific antigens are recognized by immune cells through mechanisms mediated by human leukocyte antigen.

Under pathologic chronic conditions such as in chronic diarrhea, infections, irritable bowel syndrome (IBS), or inflammatory bowel disease (IBD), defects in the intestinal barrier are thought to be the reason why gut microbiota or its components interact not just with enterocytes, dendritic cells, or intraepithelial immune cells but also with other cellular components of intestinal mucosa, so that physiologic inflammation becomes a pathologic inflammation, with the activation of all intestinal cell components.[6,9,13]

CHRONIC DIARRHEA AND GUT MICROBIOTA: WHEN INTESTINAL HOMEOSTASIS IS DISTURBED

Chronic diarrhea is characterized by the presence of diarrhea for more than 4 weeks, and it requires a different diagnostic and therapeutic work-up than acute diarrhea.[14] In developing countries, chronic diarrhea is frequently caused by chronic bacterial, mycobacterial, and parasitic infections, although functional disorders, malabsorption, and IBD are also common. In developed countries, common causes of chronic diarrhea are IBS, IBD, celiac disease, malabsorption syndromes, including lactose intolerance and small intestinal bacterial overgrowth (SIBO), or chronic infections, particularly in immune-compromised patients.[15] All these conditions have been associated directly or indirectly with gut microbiota alterations (or dysbiosis). In order to classify the involvement of gut microbiota in chronic diarrheal disorders, 3 major groups of alterations are recognized:

1. Gut microbiota alteration in the presence of infectious agents
2. Gut microbiota alteration in the presence of intestinal inflammation and damage
3. Gut microbiota alteration as the major determinant of disease without signs of intestinal inflammation or damage

In the first group, main determinants are represented by pathogens, whose mechanisms of damage have been extensively studied. It is well known that many bacterial species act through the production of toxins, including[16] *Escherichia coli, Shigella dysenteriae* (with the so-called Shiga toxin); *Clostridium perfringens* (*C perfringens* enterotoxin, a-toxin, b-toxin, and u-toxin); *Clostridium difficile* (toxins A and B), *Staphylococcus aureus* (a-hemolysin), *Bacillus cereus* (cytotoxin K and hemolysin BL), and *Aeromonas hydrophila* (aerolysin, heat-labile cytotoxins, and heat-stable cytotoxins). These toxins can cause diarrhea by different mechanisms,[16] including direct action of toxins on intestinal epithelial ion channels; indirect interaction with ion transporters; and cytotoxic, hemolytic, proinflammatory action resulting in intestinal mucosal integrity loss with reduction of normal absorptive capacity. Other studies highlight how bacterial toxins or other related substances interact with other cell types deeper within the intestinal mucosa, including neuronal cells and other mesenchymal cells, modifying their functions.[12] It is possible that pathogens can determine alterations within other populations of gut microbiota, sustaining paraphysiologic changes of intestinal homeostasis.[17–19]

The second group of alterations includes chronic disorders with multifactorial pathogenesis, such as IBD, for which it remains unclear whether gut microbiota alterations are the cause or the consequence of the disease. Both qualitative and quantitative changes of the microbial population have been described, together with an increased prevalence in selective microbial strains. Crohn disease and ulcerative colitis (UC) frequently affect intestinal areas with the highest microbial concentration, such as the terminal ileum and colon, where bacterial metabolism and fermentation processes are more intensive. Darfeuille-Michaud and colleagues[20] showed a significantly increased concentration of enteroinvasive *E coli* in the terminal ileum of patients with Crohn disease, and an increased concentration of tumor necrosis factor (TNF)-α produced by macrophage activation in response to these bacterial strains. Rodemann and colleagues[21] reported an increased number of infections by *C difficile*, increasing from 4% in 2003 to 16% in 2006, whereas Swidsinsky and colleagues[22] showed that the concentration of mucosal bacteria, particularly those adhering to the intestinal mucus and enterocytes, were higher in patients with IBD (particularly Crohn disease) compared with healthy subjects. In patients with Crohn disease, higher concentrations of anaerobes, especially *Bacteroides*, has been found in the ileum and in other segments of the colon during active disease. Frank and colleagues[23] showed a decrease in bacterial biodiversity in IBD gut microbiota with a low prevalence of Firmicutes methane-producing bacteria, an increase in Enterobacteriaceae and hydrogen-producing bacteria, and a reduction of short-chain fatty acids and epithelial trophism. Similar results were reported by Scanlan and colleagues[24] in 2008.

An additional group of alterations accounts for diseases without major signs of intestinal inflammation or damage, like IBS. Up to 84% of patients with IBS have an abnormal lactulose hydrogen breath test (LBT), suggesting the presence of SIBO.[25]

Moreover, symptoms associated with IBS (bloating, abdominal pain, and altered bowel habits) are generally similar to those associated with SIBO.[25,26] Studies based on new molecular biology techniques have highlighted significant differences in the quality, quantity, and temporal stability of gut microbiota in patients with IBS compared with healthy controls. In particular, fecal samples from patients with IBS have lower levels of coliform bacteria, Lactobacilli, and Bifidobacterium species,[27,28] and higher numbers of Clostridium species[28] and Enterobacteriaceae compared with controls.[29] Patients with diarrhea-predominant IBS had a decreased number of Lactobacillus species, whereas constipated patients with IBS showed an increase in the number of Veillonella species compared with healthy controls.[30] Gut microbiota from patients with IBS were less stable over time compared with healthy subjects, as shown by DGGE fingerprint profiles[31]; the composition of mucosa-adherent microbiota is different between patients with IBS and healthy controls, with Eubacterium rectale–Clostridium coccoides being the predominant bacterial group, accounting for 48% of the total adherent bacteria in IBS compared with 32% of healthy controls. In addition, the density of the bacterial biofilm (a layer of microorganisms that forms a coat on the surface of the intestine) was significantly larger in patients with IBS.[32] More recent data have reinforced these observations, showing that microbiota from patients with IBS and healthy controls also differed in other bacterial species including Coprococcus spp, Collinsella spp and Coprobacillus spp.[33] It can be assumed that the increasing availability of new microbiological techniques will result in increasing knowledge that may lead to new therapeutic approaches.

STUDYING GUT MICROBIOTA

The major limitation of current microbiologic methods is that the classic culture-dependent techniques can detect less than 30% of bacterial species.[34] Culturing the jejunal aspirate identifying and counting colony-forming units (CFU) is currently the gold standard in diagnosing SIBO. This method, which does not characterize the gut microbiota responsible for SIBO, is invasive; for this reason other techniques are used that are based on measuring functional alterations caused by gut microbiota. These approaches include glucose breath tests (GBTs) and LBTs, which are currently widely used in clinical practice.[35] Among them, GBT has a higher diagnostic accuracy in studies comparing breath tests with cultures.[36] Certain conditions, such as hypochlorhydria, anatomic abnormalities, or gastrointestinal motility failure, may cause SIBO and consequently malabsorption. In these cases, GBT may be useful to establish whether malabsorption is caused by SIBO. Data regarding the role of SIBO in IBS are still inconclusive, and routine screening for SIBO is not recommended. GBT and LBT are hydrogen (H_2)-based breath tests, in which the determination of hydrogen (and methane) concentration in expired air is used to assess bacterial carbohydrate metabolism. Hydrogen (and methane) is normally produced in the colon by the fermentation of residual carbohydrates by gut microbiota. In SIBO, glucose, lactulose, or other sugars (including lactose or fructose) can be fermented by bacteria in the small bowel.[37] Based on different studies and on a recent consensus conference, GBT is the breath test with the best diagnostic accuracy for diagnosing SIBO.[36]

Besides being accurate and noninvasive, H_2-breath tests have other advantages, such as lack of toxicity, low cost of substrates, and easy accessibility in clinical practice.

For the study of gut microbiota, novel and culture-independent techniques have become available that are based on the analysis of bacterial 16S rRNA or ribosomal RNA. These methods have revealed the myriad of bacterial lineages within the human gut.[34] These techniques use quantitative polymerase chain reaction, DGGE, DNA sequencing, microbial gene microarray analysis, and fluorescence in situ hybridization.[34] Major limitations of these approaches are the costs and the need for expert technologists who are able to extract, handle, and process the fecal or intestinal biopsy samples, and to interpret results. Despite intriguing experimental data, a full characterization of gut microbiota from a healthy subject is not yet possible. Furthermore, the reproducibility of results has not been studied between different centers. In addition, it is not clear whether characterization of gut microbiota should be performed on feces or on intestinal biopsies and which conditions (ie, diet, time of collection, number of samples) should be observed. Further studies are needed to provide a more robust and oriented basis for future interventional studies of microbiota modulation as a therapeutic approach for gastrointestinal and extraintestinal diseases.

GUT MICROBIOTA MODULATION

Gut microflora stability is influenced by mechanisms that directly affect gut microbiota composition as well as by mechanisms dependent on host physiology.
    Gut microbiota modulation can be achieved by:

1. Antibiotics and agents directly affecting vitality of germs
2. Probiotics: single or multiple specific bacterial or yeast species that reach the intestinal microbiota and interact with it and with gut mucosa, thereby resulting in transient gut microbiota alteration and clinical benefit to the host[38]
3. Prebiotics: substrates able to promote growth and metabolism of certain strains, thereby resulting in a transient alteration or stabilization of the gut microbiota

    Factors of host physiology that determine gut microbiota include:

1. Gastric acid secretion
2. Biliary, pancreatic, and intestinal secretion
3. Visceral motility
4. Mucosal structural integrity

    Alteration of any of these mechanisms can predispose to gut microbiota alterations (or dysbiosis). For this reason, many factors interacting with these mechanisms can modify gut microbiota homeostasis.
    For example, the widespread use of proton pump inhibitors (PPIs) has been associated with an increase of enteric infections: the hypochlorhydria induced by PPIs increases the translocation of *Salmonella typhimurium*, *Shigella flexneri*, *Campylobacter jejuni*, and enterotoxic *E coli* in enteric mucosa.[39–41] PPIs increase the infection rate of *C difficile*[42] and predispose to SIBO.[41] Motility alterations also can predispose to intestinal dysbiosis: in Parkinson disease there is an alteration of intestinal motility that correlates with a high rate of SIBO.[43] In diabetes, intestinal motility may be disturbed, thereby altering microbial composition and mucosal integrity and predisposing to bacterial overgrowth and mucosal inflammation.[44]
    Different approaches based on the control of these 4 factors can modulate gut microbiota composition. The use of prokinetics, for example, can increase intestinal motility and reduce luminal fermentations and bacterial growth[44]; diet low in carbohydrates can reduce insulin resistance and obesity, and modulate the composition of gut microbiota; the reduction of PPI use can decrease the number of pathogenic bacteria on the intestinal mucosa.[41]
    Later in this article, the focus is on agents used for modulation of gut microbiota.

Probiotics

Probiotics are microorganisms that, when administered in adequate amounts, confer health benefits to the host, especially by improving intestinal microbial balance.[38] They can provide a beneficial effect on intestinal epithelial cells in several ways. For example, some strains can block pathogen entry into epithelial cells by providing a functional and physical barrier: probiotics can increase the mucus barrier by release of mucin granules from goblet cells, maintaining intestinal permeability by increasing the intercellular integrity of apical tight junctions, for example by upregulating the expression of zonula occludens 1 (a tight junction protein) or by preventing tight junction protein redistribution and thereby stopping the passage of molecules into the lamina propria.[45–47]

Probiotic bacteria can antagonize pathogenic bacteria by reducing luminal pH, as shown in patients with UC following ingestion of VSL#3,[48] inhibiting bacterial adherence and translocation, or producing antibacterial substances like defensins and bacteriocins. The inhibitory activity of these bacteriocins varies. Some inhibit lactobacilli or related gram-positive bacteria, and some are active against a wider range of gram-positive and gram-negative bacteria and yeasts.[49]

Probiotics are also involved in the modulation of immune response and inflammation: probiotic bacteria can shape the mucosal immune system toward a noninflammatory, tolerogenic pattern through the induction of T cells with regulatory properties. Probiotics can downregulate the Th1 response and inhibit the production of proinflammatory cytokines, such as interleukin (IL)-12, TNF-α, and interferon-α by dendritic cells or increase the production of antiinflammatory cytokines, including IL-10 and transforming growth factor-β.[46]

Prebiotics

A dietary prebiotic is an ingredient that is selectively metabolized by bacteria, resulting in specific changes of the composition and/or activity of the gastrointestinal microbiota, thus conferring benefits on the health of the host.[50] By modulating gut microbiota composition through stimulation of growth or activity of a limited number of colonic bacteria, prebiotics indirectly regulate immune system activation. They favor the growth of beneficial bacteria rather than that of harmful bacteria. Prebiotics can also display direct effects on intestinal mucosa. The most used prebiotics are short-chain carbohydrates like inulin, fructo-oligosaccharides, and galacto-oligosaccharides. These compounds increase bifidobacteria and lactobacillus strains in the human colon, decrease enterococci and fusobacteria and lower fecal pH. These carbohydrates are fermented and produce short-chain fatty acids that stimulate enterocyte growth. Prebiotics decrease the levels of proinflammatory cytokines like IL-6 and TNF-α, reduce the levels of C-reactive protein (CRP), and increase phagocytosis, NK cells activity, and IL-10.[50,51]

Antibiotics

Antibiotics are usually used to fight infection by pathogens. Different antibiotic classes are used according to drug sensitivity of bacterial strains and to specific objectives. Antibiotic use can heavily alter the composition of gut microbiota, sometimes resulting in severe side effects. The widespread use of antibiotics has been blamed for increased C difficile infections.[52] However, the correct use of antibiotics is able to modulate gut microbiota and reduce the symptoms of many gastrointestinal conditions like IBS, IBD, and SIBO. The use of antibiotics in these conditions, in which a single pathogen cannot be identified as being responsible for the disease, requires a change in the current paradigm for antibiotic usage: from fighting the pathogen to modulating commensal and symbiotic bacteria.

Rifaximin, a nonabsorbable antibiotic used in IBS and SIBO, is effective in modulating gut microbiota. Several studies suggest that systemic antibiotics like quinolones and β-lactams, are responsible for the increase of harmful bacteria within the intestine, like enterococci and aerobic bacteria,[53] whereas rifaximin, because it acts mainly locally in the intestine, has been shown to reduce enterococci, *Clostridium* strains, *Bacteroides*, anaerobic cocci, and *E coli*, with no increase in bacterial resistance.[54]

GUT MICROBIOTA MODULATION IN CHRONIC DIARRHEA
Efficacy of Probiotics in IBS

Several studies and meta-analyses have shown the efficacy of probiotics in IBS, particularly the diarrhea type (**Table 1**). Probiotics are effective in reducing abdominal pain, bloating, and flatulence in IBS.[55,56]

When compared with placebo, Lactobacillus GG at a dose of 3×10^9 CFU/mL twice daily for 4 weeks is superior in relieving abdominal pain in patients with IBS[57]; Gade and colleagues[58] showed the efficacy of *Streptococcus faecium* in relieving abdominal pain and bloating; a probiotic mixture containing *Lactobacillus rhamnosus* GG, *L rhamnosus* LC705, *Bifidobacterium breve* Bb99, and *Propionibacterium freudenreichii* at a dose of 8 to 9×10^9 CFU/mL once a day for 6 months is effective in reducing abdominal pain, distension, flatulence, and borborygmi in nonconstipated patients with IBS.[59] VSL#3 mixture of bacteria twice daily (450 billion viable lyophilized bacteria) has been shown to reduce diarrhea, bloating, and flatulence in adult and pediatric patients with IBS.[60,61]

Lactobacillus-containing probiotic mixtures and *Saccharomyces boulardii* also are effective in the prevention of *C difficile* diarrhea in high-risk recipients of antibiotics.[62] *Bifidobacterium infantis* 35624 causes a significant improvement in composite and individual scores (abdominal pain/discomfort, bloating/distention, and bowel movement) compared with placebo when administered for 8 weeks at a dose of 1×10^{10} CFU.[63] Niedzielin and colleagues[64] have shown the efficacy of *Lactobacillus plantarum* 299V 5×10^7 CFU/mL twice a day for 4 weeks in reduction of abdominal pain, bowel movements, and bloating in patients with IBS. In a recent double-blind, placebo-controlled clinical trial, *Lactobacillus acidophilus* NCFM and *Bifidobacterium lactis* Bi07 twice a day at a dose of 2×10^{11} CFU/mL are more effective than placebo in improving bloating in nonconstipated patients with IBS over 8 weeks.[65] A mixture of *L acidophilus* and *Bifidobacterium bifidum* at a dose of 2.5×10^{10} CFU/mL once a day for 8 weeks significantly reduces symptom severity score and number of days with pain and improves satisfaction with bowel habits and quality of life compared with placebo.[66] Tsuchiya and colleagues[67] showed the efficacy of a mixture of *Lactobacillus helviticus* (1.25×10^6), *L acidophilus* (1.3×10^9), and *Bifidobacterium longum* (4.95×10^9) at a dose of 10 mL 3 times a day in improvement of global symptoms in nonconstipated patients with IBS. *S boulardii* at a dose of 2×10^{10}/mL once a day improves quality of life in patients with diarrhea-predominant IBS.[68]

Efficacy of Probiotics in Antibiotic-Associated Diarrhea

Several different probiotics have been evaluated in the prevention and treatment of antibiotic-associated diarrhea in adults and children, including the nonpathogenic yeast *S boulardii* and multiple lactic-acid fermenting bacteria (**Table 2**). *S boulardii* is efficacious in preventing postantibiotic diarrhea compared with placebo in patients treated with antibiotics like β-lactams[69,70]; *S boulardii* reduces the incidence of

Table 1
Probiotics in treatment of irritable bowel syndrome

Study	Probiotic	Dosage	Duration	Results
Gawronska et al[57]	Lactobacillus rhamnosus GG	3×10^9 CFU/mL bid	4 wk	Treatment success (resolution of pain and relaxed face): 33% vs 5.1% ($P = .04$); reduced frequency of pain ($P = .02$)
Kajander et al[59]	L rhamnosus GG, L rhamnosus LC705, Bifidobacterium breve Bb99 Propionibacterium freudenreichii	$8-9 \times 10^9$ CFU/mL qd	6 mo	Significant reduction in total symptom score (abdominal pain, distension, flatulence, and borborygmi) ($P<.015$)
Kim et al[60]	VSL#3 probiotic mixture	4.5×10^{11} CFU/mL bid	8 wk	Reduction in abdominal bloating ($P = .046$), no difference in other symptoms Kim et al 106 4.5 × 1011 48 (Rome II) Reduction in flatulence ($P = .011$), retardation of colonic transit ($P = .05$)
O'Mahony et al[63]	Bifidobacterium infantis 35624	1×10^{10} CFU	8 wk	Significant improvement in composite and individual scores (abdominal pain/discomfort, bloating/distention, and bowel movement difficulty) compared with placebo ($P<.05$)
Niedzielin et al[64]	Lactobacillus plantarum 299V	5×10^7 CFU/mL bid	4 wk	IBS symptom improvement (pain, constipation, diarrhea, and flatulence): 95% vs 15% ($P<.001$)
Ringel-Kulka et al[65]	Lactobacillus acidophilus NCFM and Bifidobacterium lactis Bi07	2×10^{11} CFU/mL bid	8 wk	Abdominal bloating improved with probiotics compared with placebo at 4 wk (4.10 vs 6.17, $P = .009$; change in bloating severity $P = .02$) and 8 wk (4.26 vs 5.84, $P = .06$; change in bloating severity $P<.01$
Williams et al[66]	L acidophilus and Bifidobacterium bifidum	2.5×10^{10} CFU/mL qd	8 wk	Significant reduction in symptom severity score and number of days with pain and improvement of satisfaction of bowel habit and quality of life compared with placebo ($P<.05$)
Tsuchiya at al[67]	Lactobacillus helviticus (1.25 × 106), L acidophilus (1.3 × 109) and Bifidobacterium longum (4.95 × 109)	10 mL tid	12 wk	Symptom improvement of IBS: 80% vs 10% ($P<.01$)
Choi et al[68]	Saccharomyces boulardii	2×10^{10}/mL qd	4 wk	The overall improvement in IBS-QOL higher in S boulardii group than placebo (15.4% vs 7.0%; $P<.05$)

Abbreviations: CFU, colony-forming units; QOL, quality of life.

Table 2
Probiotics in preventing antibiotics related diarrhea

Study	Probiotic	Dosage	Patients	Results
Surawicz et al[69]	S boulardii	500 mg bid	Hospitalized adults (treated with multiple antibiotics such as clindamycin, cephalosporins, or trimethoprim–sulfamethoxazole)	Decreased diarrhea: placebo 21.8% vs SB 9.5% $P = .038$
McFarland et al[70]	S boulardii	500 mg bid	Hospitalized adults treated with β-lactams	Decreased diarrhea: placebo 14.6% vs SB 7.2%; $P = .02$
Bleichner et al[72]	S boulardii	500 mg 4 tid	Adult patients in ICU being tube fed	Fewer days with diarrhea: placebo 18.9 vs 14.2 $P = .0069$
Vanderhoof et al[74]	Lactobacillus GG	1–2 × 10^{10} CFU/mL daily	Outpatient children 6 mo to 10 y	Decreased diarrhea: placebo 26% vs LGG 8% $P = $ NS
Siitonen et al[75]	Lactobacillus GG	125 mL yoghurt bid	Adult volunteers treated with erythromycin	Decreased diarrhea, flatulence
Cimperman et al[76]	Lactobacillus reuteri	1 × 10^{10} CFU/mL bid	Hospitalized adults	Significantly lower frequency of diarrhea compared with placebo in patients treated with L reuteri (50% in the placebo group vs 7.7% in the probiotic group, $P = .02$)
Ruszczyński et al[77]	L rhamnosus	2 × 10^{10} CFU/mL qd	Outpatient children 3 mo to 14 y	Decreased diarrhea: placebo 17% vs L rhamnosus 7.5%

Abbreviations: ICU, intensive care unit; LGG, Lactobacillus GG; NS, not significant; SB, Saccharomyces boulardii.

antibiotic-associated diarrhea at a dose of 200 to 1000 mg/d in hospitalized adults.[71] Bleichner and colleagues[72] showed the efficacy of S boulardii in reducing the duration of diarrhea in critically ill patients treated with antibiotics. Moreover, S boulardii is effective in preventing antibiotic-associated diarrhea in patients with Helicobacter pylori infection treated with antibiotic eradication therapy, with an increase in H pylori eradication rate.[73] Lactobacillus GG was used by Vanderhoof and colleagues[74] in the treatment of children with antibiotic-associated diarrhea, showing a significant reduction in diarrhea duration but not in frequency; another study indicated a significant reduction in flatulence and abdominal pain during antibiotic-associated diarrhea.[75] In a recent placebo-controlled pilot study, Lactobacillus reuteri 1×10^{10} twice daily for 4 weeks significantly decreased antibiotic-associated diarrhea among hospitalized adults.[76] L rhamnosus at a dose of 2×10^{10} CFU/mL once daily reduced the incidence of diarrhea in children treated with antibiotics.[77] A mixture containing Lactobacillus casei DN-114 001 (L casei imunitas) (1.0×10^8 CFU/mL), Streptococcus thermophilus (1.0×10^8 CFU/mL), and Lactobacillus bulgaricus (1.0×10^7 CFU/mL) reduces the risk of diarrhea (also C difficile diarrhea) in hospitalized patients treated with antibiotics.[78]

Efficacy of Probiotics in IBD

Probiotics have been studied in patients with IBD, in whom they have shown efficacy mainly in maintenance of remission (**Table 3**). Kruis and colleagues[79] showed that probiotic treatment with oral E coli Nissle at a dose of 200 mg/d (25×10^9 CFU/mL) for 3 months has the same efficacy in maintenance of remission in UC as mesalamine at a dose of 1200 mg/d for 3 months; these results have been confirmed by Rembacken and colleagues[80] for maintenance of remission in UC for 12 months. From these results, the European Crohn's and Colitis Organization recommends the use of E coli Nissle as an alternative to 5-aminosalicylic acid (5-ASA) for maintenance in UC.[81]

A recent study showed the efficacy of B breve and the prebiotic galacto-oligosaccharide in UC.[82] Lactobacillus GG at a dose of 18×10^9 CFU/mL once a day is as effective and safe for maintaining remission in patients with UC as mesalamine 2400 mg/d.[83] Tursi and colleagues[84] showed the efficacy of the VSL#3 probiotic mixture at the dose of 3.6×10^9 CFU/mL once a day for 8 weeks in reducing UC activity in patients affected by relapsing mild to moderate UC who are being treated with 5-ASA and/or immune-suppressants at stable doses. Furthermore, VSL#3 at a dose of 3.6 g/d is also effective in maintaining remission in patients affected by refractory pouchitis after antibiotic treatment.[85] VSL#3 is considered efficacious in the treatment as well as in the maintenance of remission of pouchitis, with a high grade of evidence.[86,87] Guslandi and colleagues[88] showed the efficacy of S boulardii 1 g daily in addition to mesalamine 1 g daily for 6 months in the maintenance of remission of Crohn disease, compared with mesalamine 1 g per day. E coli 1917 was also used in maintenance of remission of Crohn disease.[89]

No efficacy in the treatment or the maintenance of remission of patients with IBD has been shown for other probiotics, whereas some probiotics (Lactobacillus species) caused adverse effects in patients with Crohn disease.[90–92] There is not enough evidence to suggest that probiotics are beneficial for the maintenance of remission in Crohn disease.[93]

Efficacy of Antibiotics

Antibiotics are used in many gastrointestinal diseases, like SIBO, IBS, and IBD.

Table 3
Probiotics in maintenance of remission in IBD

Study	Probiotic	Dosage	Duration	Patients	Results
Kruis et al[79]	E coli strain Nissle (serotype 06: K5: H1)	200 mg/d vs mesalamine 1.2 g	12 wk	120 patients with inactive UC	No statistical differences in relapse rates between E coli and mesalazine 1200 mg (11.3% mesalazine vs 16.0% E coli Nissle 1917)
Rembacken et al[80]	E coli strain Nissle (serotype 06: K5: H1)	200 mg/d vs mesalamine 1.2 g	12 mo	120 patients with UC	No statistical differences in mean time to remission: 44 d in the mesalazine group vs 42 d in E coli group
Zocco et al[83]	Lactobacillus GG	18 × 10⁹ CFU/mL qd vs Mesalamine 2400 g/d	12 mo	187 patients with inactive UC	No difference in relapse rate at 6 (P = .44) and 12 mo (P = .77) among the 3 treatment groups
Tursi et al[84]	VSL#3 mixture	3.6 × 10⁹ CFU/mL qd vs placebo	8 wk	144 patients affected by relapsing UC already being treated with 5-aminosalicylic acid and/or immunosuppressant at stable doses	Decreased disease activity index in VSL#3 group (63.1 vs 40.8)
Guslandi et al[88]	S boulardii	1 g daily + mesalamine 1 g bid vs mesalamine 1 g 3 tid	6 mo	32 patients with Crohn disease in clinical remission	Decreased relapses (6.25% in SB group vs 37.5% in mesalamine group)
Malchow et al[89]	E coli strain Nissle (serotype 06: K5: H1)	200 mg/d	12 mo	Patients with active colonic disease on steroid tapering in remission	Decreased relapse rate in E coli group (30% vs 70%)

Efficacy of antibiotics in SIBO and IBS

Antibiotics are the cornerstone of therapy for SIBO (**Table 4**). Systemic and topical anti-biotics can be used in SIBO: the most valid antibiotic regimens used in SIBO are based on metronidazole or ciprofloxacin, with no difference in efficacy.[94] Lauritano and colleagues[95] showed the efficacy of nonabsorbable antibiotics, comparing them with a systemic antibiotic treatment of SIBO: rifaximin, a semisynthetic, rifamycin-based, nonsystemic antibiotic, with low gastrointestinal absorption and good bactericidal activity, at a dose of 1200 mg/d for 7 days was significantly superior to metronidazole 750 mg/d for 7 days. At a dose of 800 mg per day for 4 weeks, rifaximin was safe and effective in reducing symptoms in patients with SIBO of multiple causes, especially when diarrhea was the dominant symptom; and it normalized the GBT in approximately half of the patients treated.[96] Scarpellini and colleagues[97] showed that rifaximin at a dose of 1600 mg/d for 1 month is more effective than 1200 mg/d in normalizing GBT in patients with SIBO, with similar compliance and side effect profile. *Bacillus clausii* is effective in the treatment of SIBO compared with rifaximin and ciprofloxacin.[98]

Antibiotics have also been used in IBS: neomycin at a dose of 1 g/d for 10 days improved gastrointestinal symptoms in IBS (placebo controlled) and clinical response correlated with normalization of LBT.[26] Rifaximin is effective in IBS without constipation: at a dose of 550 mg 3 times daily for 2 weeks, it is more effective than placebo in controlling daily IBS symptoms.[99] A recent study by Pimentel and colleagues[100] showed the efficacy of rifaximin for 2 weeks at a dose of 550 mg 3 times a day in patients with IBS without constipation in reducing diarrhea, bloating. and abdominal pain. Jolley[101] showed that rifaximin at a dose of 2400 mg/d improves IBS symptoms in patients not responding to 1200 mg/d. Rifaximin at a dose of 400 mg 3 times daily for 10 days improves IBS symptoms for up to 10 weeks after the discontinuation of therapy.[102] The usefulness of rifaximin in the treatment of intestinal inflammation was recently shown, and this was linked to the effect of rifaximin through human pregnenolone X receptor–mediated inhibition of the nuclear factor (NF)-κB signaling cascade.[103]

Efficacy of antibiotics in IBD

Antibiotics have been used in IBD for inducing and maintaining remission (**Table 5**). When used in mild to moderate flare-ups of Crohn disease, ciprofloxacin at a dose of 1 g daily has similar efficacy to mesalazine at a dose of 4 g/d, with a response rate of 40% to 50% after 6 weeks.[104] Ciprofloxacin is efficacious in increasing the remission rate of perianal fistulizing Crohn disease.[105]

In a 16-week crossover trial, metronidazole was as effective as sulfasalazine in inducing remission in moderate Crohn disease.[106] The combination of ciprofloxacin and metronidazole has been compared with steroids, showing 46% versus 63% remission.[107] Metronidazole (250 mg twice a day) plus ciprofloxacin (200 mg 3 times daily) for 4 weeks is efficient for reducing CRP levels and disease activity index in active Crohn disease.[108] A recent study showed the effect of an 8-week course of metronidazole and azithromycin in inducing clinical remission in mild to moderate Crohn disease in children and young adults.[109]

The combination of antimycobacterial agents clarithromycin (750 mg/d), rifabutin (450 mg/d), and clofazimine (50 mg/d) was not superior to placebo in inducing remission in active Crohn disease during 2 years of therapy.[110] The lack of adequate studies precludes the routine use of antibiotics that are only considered appropriate for septic complications, symptoms attributable to bacterial overgrowth, or perianal disease in active Crohn disease, whereas there is no evidence for the maintenance of medically induced remission.[93]

Table 4
Antibiotics in treatment of IBS and SIBO

Study	Antibiotic and Dosages	Duration	Patients	Results
Castiglione et al[94]	Metronidazole (250 mg 3 times daily) vs ciprofloxacin (500 mg bid) vs placebo	10 d	29 patients with CD with SIBO	In both groups antibiotic treatment improved intestinal symptoms: bloating (85% and 83%), stool softness (44% and 50%), abdominal pain (50% and 43%)
Lauritano et al[95]	Rifaximin 1200 mg/d vs metronidazole 750 mg/d	7 d	142 patients with SIBO	GBT normalization rate significantly higher in the rifaximin than metronidazole group (63.4% vs 43.7%; P<.05)
Scarpellini et al[97]	Rifaximin 1600 mg/d vs rifaximin 1200 mg/d	7 d	80 patients with SIBO	GBT normalization rate significantly higher with rifaximin 1600 mg/d than 1200 mg/d (80% vs 58%; P<.05) with the same side effects
Pimentel et al[100]	Rifaximin 550 mg 3 tid vs placebo	2 wk + 10 wk of FU	1260 patients with IBS without constipation	More patients in the rifaximin group than in the placebo group had adequate relief of global IBS symptoms during the first 4 wk after treatment (40.8% vs 31.2%, P = .01)
Jolley[101]	Rifaximin 2400 mg/d	10 d	81 patients with IBS without constipation not responders to rifaximin 120 mg/d for 10 d	Improvement in IBS symptoms in 53% of nonresponders to 1200 mg/d rifaximin

Abbreviations: CD, Crohn disease; FU, follow-up.

Table 5
Antibiotics in IBD

Study	Antibiotic and Dosages	Duration	Patients	Results
Colombel et al[104]	Ciprofloxacin 1 g/d vs mesalazine 4 g/d	6 wk	30 patients with a mild to moderate flare-up of Crohn disease (mean Crohn Disease Activity Index 217)	Complete remission was observed in 56% of ciprofloxacin group and 55% in mesalazine group
Prantera et al[107]	Ciprofloxacin 500 mg bid + metronidazole 1000 mg/d vs methylprednisolone 0.7–1 mg/kg/d	12 wk	41 patients with active Crohn disease	No inferiority of antibiotics in remission compared with steroids (NS)
Rutgeers et al[111]	Metronidazole (20 mg/kg) vs placebo	12 wk	60 patients with CD had curative ileal resection and primary anastomosis during the first week	The incidence of severe endoscopic recurrence was significantly reduced by metronidazole (3 of 23; 13%) compared with placebo (12 of 28; 43%; $P = .02$)
D'Haens et al[112]	Metronidazole 250 mg 3 tid + AZA 150 mg/d vs AZA 150 mg/d + placebo	1 y	81 patients with CD with ileocecal resection	Significant endoscopic recurrence in 44% of patients in the metronidazole/AZA group and in 69% of patients in the AZA/placebo group
Uehara et al[115]	Amoxicillin 500 mg 3 tid, tetracycline 500 mg 3 times a day, and metronidazole 250 mg 3 times a day	1 y	25 patients with active UC including 17 steroid-dependent or refractory cases	CAI and endoscopic scores significantly decreased compared with those before treatment after antibiotics also in steroid refractory or dependent UC
Turunen et al[116]	Ciprofloxacin 500–750 mg bid	6 mo	83 patients with UC in maintenance treatment with mesalamine and tapering steroid	Treatment failure rate 21% in the ciprofloxacin-treated group and 44% in the placebo group ($P = .02$)
Shen et al[117]	Ciprofloxacin 1000 mg/d vs metronidazole 20 mg/kg/d	2 wk	16 patients with acute pouchitis	Significantly greater reduction in the ciprofloxacin group than in the metronidazole group in the total PDAI (6.9 ± 1.2 vs 3.8 ± 1.7; $P = .002$), symptom score (2.4 ± 0.9 vs 1.3 ± 0.9; $P = .03$), and endoscopic score (3.6 ± 1.3 vs 1.9 ± 1.5; $P = .03$)
Shen et al[118]	Ciprofloxacin 1 g/d and tinidazole 15 mg/kg/d	4 wk	16 Patients with UC with chronic refractory pouchitis	Patients taking ciprofloxacin and tinidazole had a significant reduction in total PDAI scores and subscores and a significant improvement in quality-of-life scores ($P<.002$)

Abbreviations: AZA, Azathioprine; CAI, Colitis Activity Index; PDAI, Pouchitis Disease Activity Index.

Antibiotics are effective for the prevention of postoperative recurrence: metronidazole at a dose of 20 mg/kg for 3 months after surgery significantly reduces the incidence of severe endoscopic recurrence during 1 year of follow-up.[111] The combination of metronidazole and azathioprine has been shown to lower endoscopic recurrence rates and decrease severity of recurrences 12 months after surgery, predicting a more favorable clinical outcome.[112] Ornidazol, another nitroimidazol antibiotic, at a dose of 1 g daily for 1 year, was effective for the prevention of clinical and endoscopic recurrence of Crohn disease after ileocolonic resection, but side effects were important.[113]

The effect of antibiotics for inducing and maintaining remission in UC is limited: antibiotics as an adjunct to steroids do not modify the outcome of severe colitis.[45–48] Triple therapy with amoxicillin (500 mg/d), tetracycline (500 mg/d), and metronidazole (250 mg 3 times daily) for 2 weeks has been shown to be safe and effective in reducing clinical activity and endoscopic and histologic scores after 14 months of follow-up.[114] A recent study proved the efficacy of this triple antibiotic therapy at higher doses (amoxicillin 500 mg 3 times a day, tetracycline 500 mg 3 times a day, and metronidazole 250 mg 3 times a day) in severe, refractory, and steroid-dependent UC.[115] The addition of ciprofloxacin (500–750 mg daily for 6 months) to conventional therapy with mesalazine and prednisone reduces the treatment failure rate.[116] The lack of appropriate strong clinical trials, despite evidence of efficacy, precludes the routine use of antibiotics for inducing and maintaining remission in UC.[81]

Antibiotics are the mainstay of treatment of acute and chronic pouchitis; metronidazole and ciprofloxacin are the most frequently used. A 2-week course of ciprofloxacin (1000 mg/d) or metronidazole (20 mg/kg/d) is effective in the treatment of acute pouchitis with significant reduction in Pouchitis Activity Index compared with placebo; ciprofloxacin is associated with a larger reduction of pouchitis disease activity and is better tolerated.[117] Ciprofloxacin (1000 mg/d) is also effective in chronic refractory pouchitis when added to tinidazole (15 mg/kg/d).[118] Combined therapy with ciprofloxacin (500 mg twice a day) and rifaximin (2 g daily) for 2 weeks is effective in active chronic refractory pouchitis.[119]

SUMMARY

This article presents the crucial importance of gut microbiota as an organ of the human body. It describes major alterations in the course of chronic diarrhea associated with pathogens. The major limitation of current studies is that the characterization of gut microbiota is not possible with currently available routine examinations. More precise (and considerably more expensive) technologies would help in doing this, but until now they have not been available for large clinical trials. In addition, gut microbiota have not been characterized in normal subjects. In chronic inflammatory conditions, in particular, modifications of gut microbiota coexist with immunologic alterations of the host.

Studies assessing the clinical efficacy of probiotics and prebiotics have followed rules that are different from the currently acceptable rules for the study of drug effects, which is the main reason why it is likely that the real efficacy of probiotics and prebiotics in modulating gut microbiota functions is probably underestimated or misestimated. Dose findings studies or studies evaluating the mechanisms of action of different strains of probiotics or different types of prebiotics have been performed very rarely.

It is hoped that this review will encourage gastroenterologists to pursue gut microbiota research to better understand the physiology and pathology of gut microbiota homeostasis.

ACKNOWLEDGMENT

The authors acknowledge Fondazione Ricerca In Medicina ONLUS, Bologna, Italy.

REFERENCES

1. Damman CJ, Surawicz CM. comment to: "the gut microbiota: a microbial arsenal protecting us from infectious and radiation-induced diarrhea" by Sekirov I, Tam NM, Jogova M, et al. Infect Immun 2008;76:4726–36. Gastroenterology 2009;136(2):722–4.
2. Backhed F, Ley RE, Sonnenburg JL, et al. Host-bacterial mutualism in the human intestine. Science 2005;307(5717):1915–20.
3. Zoetendal EG, Rajilic-Stojanovic M, de Vos WM. High-throughput diversity and functionality analysis of the gastrointestinal tract microbiota. Gut 2008;57(11): 1605–15.
4. Eckburg PB, Bik EM, Bernstein CN, et al. Diversity of the human intestinal microbial flora. Science 2005;308(5728):1635–8.
5. Guarner F. Enteric flora in health and disease. Digestion 2006;73(Suppl 1):5–12.
6. Sartor RB. Microbial influences in inflammatory bowel diseases. Gastroenterology 2008;134(2):577–94.
7. Flint HJ, Bayer EA, Rincon MT, et al. Polysaccharide utilization by gut bacteria: potential for new insights from genomic analysis. Nat Rev Microbiol 2008;6(2): 121–31.
8. Backhed F, Manchester JK, Semenkovich CF, et al. Mechanisms underlying the resistance to diet-induced obesity in germ-free mice. Proc Natl Acad Sci U S A 2007;104(3):979–84.
9. Fiocchi C. What is "physiological" intestinal inflammation and how does it differ from "pathological" inflammation? Inflamm Bowel Dis 2008;14(Suppl 2):S77–8.
10. Scaldaferri F, Fiocchi C. Inflammatory bowel disease: progress and current concepts of etiopathogenesis. J Dig Dis 2007;8(4):171–8.
11. Payne CM, Fass R, Bernstein H, et al. Pathogenesis of diarrhea in the adult: diagnostic challenges and life-threatening conditions. Eur J Gastroenterol Hepatol 2006;18(10):1047–51.
12. Wood JD. Effects of bacteria on the enteric nervous system: implications for the irritable bowel syndrome. J Clin Gastroenterol 2007;41(Suppl 1):S7–19.
13. Packey CD, Sartor RB. Commensal bacteria, traditional and opportunistic pathogens, dysbiosis and bacterial killing in inflammatory bowel diseases. Curr Opin Infect Dis 2009;22(3):292–301.
14. Donowitz M, Kokke FT, Saidi R. Evaluation of patients with chronic diarrhea. N Engl J Med 1995;332(11):725–9.
15. American Gastroenterological Association medical position statement: guidelines for the evaluation and management of chronic diarrhea. Gastroenterology 1999;116(6):1461–3.
16. Laohachai KN, Bahadi R, Hardo MB, et al. The role of bacterial and nonbacterial toxins in the induction of changes in membrane transport: implications for diarrhea. Toxicon 2003;42(7):687–707.
17. Tomasello G, Bellavia M, Palumbo VD, et al. From gut microflora imbalance to mycobacteria infection: is there a relationship with chronic intestinal inflammatory diseases? Ann Ital Chir 2011;82(5):361–8.
18. de Sablet T, Chassard C, Bernalier-Donadille A, et al. Human microbiota-secreted factors inhibit Shiga toxin synthesis by enterohemorrhagic *Escherichia coli* O157:H7. Infect Immun 2009;77(2):783–90.

19. Endt K, Stecher B, Chaffron S, et al. The microbiota mediates pathogen clearance from the gut lumen after non-typhoidal *Salmonella* diarrhea. PLoS Pathog 2010;6(9):e1001097.

20. Darfeuille-Michaud A, Boudeau J, Bulois P, et al. High prevalence of adherent-invasive *Escherichia coli* associated with ileal mucosa in Crohn's disease. Gastroenterology 2004;127(2):412–21.

21. Rodemann JF, Dubberke ER, Reske KA, et al. Incidence of *Clostridium difficile* infection in inflammatory bowel disease. Clin Gastroenterol Hepatol 2007;5(3): 339–44.

22. Swidsinski A, Ladhoff A, Pernthaler A, et al. Mucosal flora in inflammatory bowel disease. Gastroenterology 2002;122(1):44–54.

23. Frank DN, St Amand AL, Feldman RA, et al. Molecular-phylogenetic characterization of microbial community imbalances in human inflammatory bowel diseases. Proc Natl Acad Sci U S A 2007;104(34):13780–5.

24. Scanlan PD, Marchesi JR. Micro-eukaryotic diversity of the human distal gut microbiota: qualitative assessment using culture-dependent and -independent analysis of faeces. ISME J 2008;2(12):1183–93.

25. Pimentel M, Chow EJ, Lin HC. Eradication of small intestinal bacterial overgrowth reduces symptoms of irritable bowel syndrome. Am J Gastroenterol 2000;95(12):3503–6.

26. Pimentel M, Chow EJ, Lin HC. Normalization of lactulose breath testing correlates with symptom improvement in irritable bowel syndrome. a double-blind, randomized, placebo-controlled study. Am J Gastroenterol 2003;98(2): 412–9.

27. Si JM, Yu YC, Fan YJ, et al. Intestinal microecology and quality of life in irritable bowel syndrome patients. World J Gastroenterol 2004;10(12):1802–5.

28. Matto J, Maunuksela L, Kajander K, et al. Composition and temporal stability of gastrointestinal microbiota in irritable bowel syndrome–a longitudinal study in IBS and control subjects. FEMS Immunol Med Microbiol 2005;43(2): 213–22.

29. Bradley HK, Wyatt GM, Bayliss CE, et al. Instability in the faecal flora of a patient suffering from food-related irritable bowel syndrome. J Med Microbiol 1987; 23(1):29–32.

30. Malinen E, Rinttila T, Kajander K, et al. Analysis of the fecal microbiota of irritable bowel syndrome patients and healthy controls with real-time PCR. Am J Gastroenterol 2005;100(2):373–82.

31. Maukonen J, Matto J, Satokari R, et al. PCR DGGE and RT-PCR DGGE show diversity and short-term temporal stability in the *Clostridium coccoides-Eubacterium rectale* group in the human intestinal microbiota. FEMS Microbiol Ecol 2006;58(3):517–28.

32. Swidsinski A, Weber J, Loening-Baucke V, et al. Spatial organization and composition of the mucosal flora in patients with inflammatory bowel disease. J Clin Microbiol 2005;43(7):3380–9.

33. Kassinen A, Krogius-Kurikka L, Makivuokko H, et al. The fecal microbiota of irritable bowel syndrome patients differs significantly from that of healthy subjects. Gastroenterology 2007;133(1):24–33.

34. Suau A, Bonnet R, Sutren M, et al. Direct analysis of genes encoding 16S rRNA from complex communities reveals many novel molecular species within the human gut. Appl Environ Microbiol 1999;65(11):4799–807.

35. Bures J, Cyrany J, Kohoutova D, et al. Small intestinal bacterial overgrowth syndrome. World J Gastroenterol 2010;16(24):2978–90.

36. Gasbarrini A, Corazza GR, Gasbarrini G, et al. Methodology and indications of H2-breath testing in gastrointestinal diseases: the Rome Consensus Conference. Aliment Pharmacol Ther 2009;29(Suppl 1):1–49.

37. Levitt MD. Production and excretion of hydrogen gas in man. N Engl J Med 1969;281(3):122–7.

38. FAO/WHO. Probiotics in food. Health and nutritional properties and guidelines for evaluation. Rome: FAO Food and Nutrition Paper; 2006. p. 85.

39. Laine L, Ahnen D, McClain C, et al. Review article: potential gastrointestinal effects of long-term acid suppression with proton pump inhibitors. Aliment Pharmacol Ther 2000;14(6):651–68.

40. Neal KR, Scott HM, Slack RC, et al. Omeprazole as a risk factor for campylobacter gastroenteritis: case-control study. BMJ 1996;312(7028):414–5.

41. Williams C, McColl KE. Review article: proton pump inhibitors and bacterial overgrowth. Aliment Pharmacol Ther 2006;23(1):3–10.

42. Dial S, Alrasadi K, Manoukian C, et al. Risk of *Clostridium difficile* diarrhea among hospital inpatients prescribed proton pump inhibitors: cohort and case-control studies. CMAJ 2004;171(1):33–8.

43. Gabrielli M, Bonazzi P, Scarpellini E, et al. Prevalence of small intestinal bacterial overgrowth in Parkinson's disease. Mov Disord 2011;26(5):889–92.

44. Burcelin R, Serino M, Chabo C, et al. Gut microbiota and diabetes: from pathogenesis to therapeutic perspective. Acta Diabetol 2011;48(4):257–73.

45. Gareau MG, Sherman PM, Walker WA. Probiotics and the gut microbiota in intestinal health and disease. Nat Rev Gastroenterol Hepatol 2010;7(9):503–14.

46. Ng SC, Hart AL, Kamm MA, et al. Mechanisms of action of probiotics: recent advances. Inflamm Bowel Dis 2009;15(2):300–10.

47. Otte JM, Podolsky DK. Functional modulation of enterocytes by gram-positive and gram-negative microorganisms. Am J Physiol Gastrointest Liver Physiol 2004;286(4):G613–26.

48. Venturi A, Gionchetti P, Rizzello F, et al. Impact on the composition of the faecal flora by a new probiotic preparation: preliminary data on maintenance treatment of patients with ulcerative colitis. Aliment Pharmacol Ther 1999;13(8):1103–8.

49. Nemcova R. Criteria for selection of lactobacilli for probiotic use. Vet Med (Praha) 1997;42(1):19–27 [in Slovak].

50. Roberfroid M, Gibson GR, Hoyles L, et al. Prebiotic effects: metabolic and health benefits. Br J Nutr 2010;104(Suppl 2):S1–63.

51. Macfarlane S, Macfarlane GT, Cummings JH. Review article: prebiotics in the gastrointestinal tract. Aliment Pharmacol Ther 2006;24(5):701–14.

52. Khanna S, Pardi DS. The growing incidence and severity of *Clostridium difficile* infection in inpatient and outpatient settings. Expert Rev Gastroenterol Hepatol 2010;4(4):409–16.

53. Sullivan A, Edlund C, Nord CE. Effect of antimicrobial agents on the ecological balance of human microflora. Lancet Infect Dis 2001;1(2):101–14.

54. Scarpignato C, Pelosini I. Experimental and clinical pharmacology of rifaximin, a gastrointestinal selective antibiotic. Digestion 2006;73(Suppl 1):13–27.

55. Hoveyda N, Heneghan C, Mahtani KR, et al. A systematic review and meta-analysis: probiotics in the treatment of irritable bowel syndrome. BMC Gastroenterol 2009;9:15.

56. Ki Cha B, Mun Jung S, Hwan Choi C, et al. The effect of a multispecies probiotic mixture on the symptoms and fecal microbiota in diarrhea-dominant irritable bowel syndrome: a randomized, double-blind, placebo-controlled trial. J Clin Gastroenterol 2012;46(3):220–7.

57. Gawronska A, Dziechciarz P, Horvath A, et al. A randomized double-blind placebo-controlled trial of Lactobacillus GG for abdominal pain disorders in children. Aliment Pharmacol Ther 2007;25(2):177–84.

58. Gade J, Thorn P. Paraghurt for patients with irritable bowel syndrome. A controlled clinical investigation from general practice. Scand J Prim Health Care 1989;7(1):23–6.

59. Kajander K, Hatakka K, Poussa T, et al. A probiotic mixture alleviates symptoms in irritable bowel syndrome patients: a controlled 6-month intervention. Aliment Pharmacol Ther 2005;22(5):387–94.

60. Kim HJ, Vazquez Roque MI, Camilleri M, et al. A randomized controlled trial of a probiotic combination VSL# 3 and placebo in irritable bowel syndrome with bloating. Neurogastroenterol Motil 2005;17(5):687–96.

61. Guandalini S, Magazzu G, Chiaro A, et al. VSL#3 improves symptoms in children with irritable bowel syndrome: a multicenter, randomized, placebo-controlled, double-blind, crossover study. J Pediatr Gastroenterol Nutr 2010;51(1):24–30.

62. Na X, Kelly C. Probiotics in *Clostridium difficile* infection. J Clin Gastroenterol 2011;45(Suppl):S154–8.

63. O'Mahony L, McCarthy J, Kelly P, et al. *Lactobacillus* and *Bifidobacterium* in irritable bowel syndrome: symptom responses and relationship to cytokine profiles. Gastroenterology 2005;128(3):541–51.

64. Niedzielin K, Kordecki H, Birkenfeld B. A controlled, double-blind, randomized study on the efficacy of *Lactobacillus plantarum* 299V in patients with irritable bowel syndrome. Eur J Gastroenterol Hepatol 2001;13(10):1143–7.

65. Ringel-Kulka T, Palsson OS, Maier D, et al. Probiotic bacteria *Lactobacillus acidophilus* NCFM and *Bifidobacterium lactis* Bi-07 versus placebo for the symptoms of bloating in patients with functional bowel disorders: a double-blind study. J Clin Gastroenterol 2011;45(6):518–25.

66. Williams EA, Stimpson J, Wang D, et al. Clinical trial: a multistrain probiotic preparation significantly reduces symptoms of irritable bowel syndrome in a double-blind placebo-controlled study. Aliment Pharmacol Ther 2009;29(1):97–103.

67. Tsuchiya J, Barreto R, Okura R, et al. Single-blind follow-up study on the effectiveness of a symbiotic preparation in irritable bowel syndrome. Chin J Dig Dis 2004;5(4):169–74.

68. Choi CH, Jo SY, Park HJ, et al. A randomized, double-blind, placebo-controlled multicenter trial of *Saccharomyces boulardii* in irritable bowel syndrome: effect on quality of life. J Clin Gastroenterol 2011;45(8):679–83.

69. Surawicz CM, Elmer GW, Speelman P, et al. Prevention of antibiotic-associated diarrhea by *Saccharomyces boulardii*: a prospective study. Gastroenterology 1989;96(4):981–8.

70. McFarland LV, Surawicz CM, Greenberg RN, et al. Prevention of beta-lactam-associated diarrhea by *Saccharomyces boulardii* compared with placebo. Am J Gastroenterol 1995;90(3):439–48.

71. Can M, Besirbellioglu BA, Avci IY, et al. Prophylactic *Saccharomyces boulardii* in the prevention of antibiotic-associated diarrhea: a prospective study. Med Sci Monit 2006;12(4):PI19–22.

72. Bleichner G, Blehaut H, Mentec H, et al. *Saccharomyces boulardii* prevents diarrhea in critically ill tube-fed patients. A multicenter, randomized, double-blind placebo-controlled trial. Intensive Care Med 1997;23(5):517–23.

73. Cremonini F, Di Caro S, Covino M, et al. Effect of different probiotic preparations on anti-*Helicobacter pylori* therapy-related side effects: a parallel group, triple blind, placebo-controlled study. Am J Gastroenterol 2002;97(11):2744–9.

74. Vanderhoof JA, Whitney DB, Antonson DL, et al. Lactobacillus GG in the prevention of antibiotic-associated diarrhea in children. J Pediatr 1999;135(5): 564–8.

75. Siitonen S, Vapaatalo H, Salminen S, et al. Effect of Lactobacillus GG yoghurt in prevention of antibiotic associated diarrhoea. Ann Med 1990;22(1):57–9.

76. Cimperman L, Bayless G, Best K, et al. A randomized, double-blind, placebo-controlled pilot study of *Lactobacillus reuteri* ATCC 55730 for the prevention of antibiotic-associated diarrhea in hospitalized adults. J Clin Gastroenterol 2011;45(9):785–9.

77. Ruszczynski M, Radzikowski A, Szajewska H. Clinical trial: effectiveness of *Lactobacillus rhamnosus* (strains E/N, Oxy and Pen) in the prevention of antibiotic-associated diarrhoea in children. Aliment Pharmacol Ther 2008; 28(1):154–61.

78. Hickson M, D'Souza AL, Muthu N, et al. Use of probiotic *Lactobacillus* preparation to prevent diarrhoea associated with antibiotics: randomised double blind placebo controlled trial. BMJ 2007;335(7610):80.

79. Kruis W, Schutz E, Fric P, et al. Double-blind comparison of an oral *Escherichia coli* preparation and mesalazine in maintaining remission of ulcerative colitis. Aliment Pharmacol Ther 1997;11(5):853–8.

80. Rembacken BJ, Snelling AM, Hawkey PM, et al. Non-pathogenic *Escherichia coli* versus mesalazine for the treatment of ulcerative colitis: a randomised trial. Lancet 1999;354(9179):635–9.

81. Travis SP, Stange EF, Lemann M, et al. European evidence-based consensus on the management of ulcerative colitis: current management. J Crohns Colitis 2008;2(1):24–62.

82. Ishikawa H, Matsumoto S, Ohashi Y, et al. Beneficial effects of probiotic bifidobacterium and galacto-oligosaccharide in patients with ulcerative colitis: a randomized controlled study. Digestion 2011;84(2):128–33.

83. Zocco MA, Dal Verme LZ, Cremonini F, et al. Efficacy of Lactobacillus GG in maintaining remission of ulcerative colitis. Aliment Pharmacol Ther 2006; 23(11):1567–74.

84. Tursi A, Brandimarte G, Papa A, et al. Treatment of relapsing mild-to-moderate ulcerative colitis with the probiotic VSL#3 as adjunctive to a standard pharmaceutical treatment: a double-blind, randomized, placebo-controlled study. Am J Gastroenterol 2010;105(10):2218–27.

85. Gionchetti P, Rizzello F, Venturi A, et al. Oral bacteriotherapy as maintenance treatment in patients with chronic pouchitis: a double-blind, placebo-controlled trial. Gastroenterology 2000;119(2):305–9.

86. Holubar SD, Cima RR, Sandborn WJ, et al. Treatment and prevention of pouchitis after ileal pouch-anal anastomosis for chronic ulcerative colitis. Cochrane Database Syst Rev 2010;(6):CD001176.

87. Gionchetti P, Rizzello F, Morselli C, et al. High-dose probiotics for the treatment of active pouchitis. Dis Colon Rectum 2007;50(12):2075–82 [discussion: 2082–4].

88. Guslandi M, Mezzi G, Sorghi M, et al. *Saccharomyces boulardii* in maintenance treatment of Crohn's disease. Dig Dis Sci 2000;45(7):1462–4.

89. Malchow HA. Crohn's disease and *Escherichia coli*. A new approach in therapy to maintain remission of colonic Crohn's disease? J Clin Gastroenterol 1997; 25(4):653–8.

90. Rolfe VE, Fortun PJ, Hawkey CJ, et al. Probiotics for maintenance of remission in Crohn's disease. Cochrane Database Syst Rev 2006;(4):CD004826.

91. Van Gossum A, Dewit O, Louis E, et al. Multicenter randomized-controlled clinical trial of probiotics (*Lactobacillus johnsonii*, LA1) on early endoscopic recurrence of Crohn's disease after ileo-caecal resection. Inflamm Bowel Dis 2007; 13(2):135–42.

92. Rahimi R, Nikfar S, Rahimi F, et al. A meta-analysis on the efficacy of probiotics for maintenance of remission and prevention of clinical and endoscopic relapse in Crohn's disease. Dig Dis Sci 2008;53(9):2524–31.

93. Dignass A, Van Assche G, Lindsay JO, et al. The second European evidence-based consensus on the diagnosis and management of Crohn's disease: current management. J Crohns Colitis 2010;4(1):28–62.

94. Castiglione F, Rispo A, Di Girolamo E, et al. Antibiotic treatment of small bowel bacterial overgrowth in patients with Crohn's disease. Aliment Pharmacol Ther 2003;18(11–12):1107–12.

95. Lauritano EC, Gabrielli M, Scarpellini E, et al. Antibiotic therapy in small intestinal bacterial overgrowth: rifaximin versus metronidazole. Eur Rev Med Pharmacol Sci 2009;13(2):111–6.

96. Majewski M, Reddymasu SC, Sostarich S, et al. Efficacy of rifaximin, a nonabsorbed oral antibiotic, in the treatment of small intestinal bacterial overgrowth. Am J Med Sci 2007;333(5):266–70.

97. Scarpellini E, Gabrielli M, Lauritano CE, et al. High dosage rifaximin for the treatment of small intestinal bacterial overgrowth. Aliment Pharmacol Ther 2007; 25(7):781–6.

98. Gabrielli M, Lauritano EC, Scarpellini E, et al. *Bacillus clausii* as a treatment of small intestinal bacterial overgrowth. Am J Gastroenterol 2009;104(5):1327–8.

99. Schey R, Rao SS. The role of rifaximin therapy in patients with irritable bowel syndrome without constipation. Expert Rev Gastroenterol Hepatol 2011;5(4): 461–4.

100. Pimentel M, et al. Rifaximin therapy for patients with irritable bowel syndrome without constipation. N Engl J Med 2011;364(1):22–32.

101. Jolley J. High-dose rifaximin treatment alleviates global symptoms of irritable bowel syndrome. Clin Exp Gastroenterol 2011;4:43–8.

102. Pimentel M, Park S, Mirocha J, et al. The effect of a nonabsorbed oral antibiotic (rifaximin) on the symptoms of the irritable bowel syndrome: a randomized trial. Ann Intern Med 2006;145(8):557–63.

103. Cheng J, Shah YM, Ma X, et al. Therapeutic role of rifaximin in inflammatory bowel disease: clinical implication of human pregnane X receptor activation. J Pharmacol Exp Ther 2010;335(1):32–41.

104. Colombel JF, Lemann M, Cassagnou M, et al. A controlled trial comparing ciprofloxacin with mesalazine for the treatment of active Crohn's disease. Groupe d'Etudes Therapeutiques des Affections Inflammatoires Digestives (GETAID). Am J Gastroenterol 1999;94(3):674–8.

105. Thia KT, Mahadevan U, Feagan BG, et al. Ciprofloxacin or metronidazole for the treatment of perianal fistulas in patients with Crohn's disease: a randomized, double-blind, placebo-controlled pilot study. Inflamm Bowel Dis 2009;15(1): 17–24.

106. Ursing B, Alm T, Barany F, et al. A comparative study of metronidazole and sulfasalazine for active Crohn's disease: the cooperative Crohn's disease study in Sweden. II. Result. Gastroenterology 1982;83(3):550–62.

107. Prantera C, Zannoni F, Scribano ML, et al. An antibiotic regimen for the treatment of active Crohn's disease: a randomized, controlled clinical trial of metronidazole plus ciprofloxacin. Am J Gastroenterol 1996;91(2):328–32.

108. Ishikawa T, Okamura S, Oshimoto H, et al. Metronidazole plus ciprofloxacin therapy for active Crohn's disease. Intern Med 2003;42(4):318–21.

109. Levine A, Turner D. Combined azithromycin and metronidazole therapy is effective in inducing remission in pediatric Crohn's disease. J Crohns Colitis 2011; 5(3):222–6.

110. Selby W, Pavli P, Crotty B, et al. Two-year combination antibiotic therapy with clarithromycin, rifabutin, and clofazimine for Crohn's disease. Gastroenterology 2007;132(7):2313–9.

111. Rutgeerts P, Hiele M, Geboes K, et al. Controlled trial of metronidazole treatment for prevention of Crohn's recurrence after ileal resection. Gastroenterology 1995; 108(6):1617–21.

112. D'Haens GR, Vermeire S, Van Assche G, et al. Therapy of metronidazole with azathioprine to prevent postoperative recurrence of Crohn's disease: a controlled randomized trial. Gastroenterology 2008;135(4):1123–9.

113. Rutgeerts P, Van Assche G, Vermeire S, et al. Ornidazole for prophylaxis of postoperative Crohn's disease recurrence: a randomized, double-blind, placebo-controlled trial. Gastroenterology 2005;128(4):856–61.

114. Ohkusa T, Nomura T, Terai T, et al. Effectiveness of antibiotic combination therapy in patients with active ulcerative colitis: a randomized, controlled pilot trial with long-term follow-up. Scand J Gastroenterol 2005;40(11):1334–42.

115. Uehara T, Kato K, Ohkusa T, et al. Efficacy of antibiotic combination therapy in patients with active ulcerative colitis, including refractory or steroid-dependent cases. J Gastroenterol Hepatol 2010;25(Suppl 1):S62–6.

116. Turunen UM, Farkkila MA, Hakala K, et al. Long-term treatment of ulcerative colitis with ciprofloxacin: a prospective, double-blind, placebo-controlled study. Gastroenterology 1998;115(5):1072–8.

117. Shen B, Achkar JP, Lashner BA, et al. A randomized clinical trial of ciprofloxacin and metronidazole to treat acute pouchitis. Inflamm Bowel Dis 2001;7(4):301–5.

118. Shen B, Fazio VW, Remzi FH, et al. Combined ciprofloxacin and tinidazole therapy in the treatment of chronic refractory pouchitis. Dis Colon Rectum 2007;50(4):498–508.

119. Gionchetti P, Rizzello F, Venturi A, et al. Antibiotic combination therapy in patients with chronic, treatment-resistant pouchitis. Aliment Pharmacol Ther 1999;13(6):713–8.

Diarrhea Caused By Circulating Agents

Elisabeth Fabian, PhD, Patrizia Kump, MD,
Guenter J. Krejs, MD, AGAF*

KEYWORDS

- Secretory diarrhea • Endocrine diarrhea • Pancreatic cholera • Carcinoid syndrome
- Neuroendocrine tumors

KEY POINTS

- Circulating agents reach intestinal epithelial cells and change water and electrolyte absorption to secretion.
- In Verner-Morrison syndrome (also known as pancreatic cholera or watery diarrhea, hypokalemia, hypochlorhydria [WDHH] syndrome), vasoactive intestinal polypeptide (VIP) released from a neuroendocrine tumor causes secretory diarrhea. The syndrome can be mimicked by intravenous VIP infusion in healthy subjects.
- In malignant carcinoid syndrome, secretory diarrhea is accompanied by flushing, right-sided endocardial fibrosis and sometimes bronchospasm.
- In Zollinger-Ellison syndrome (ZES), high levels of circulating gastrin lead to many liters of gastric secretions per day, a volume that overwhelms the absorptive capacity of the intestine and results in diarrhea.
- In many of the endocrine diarrhea syndromes, a somatostatin analog is capable of reducing diarrhea by decreasing the release of hormones and other tumor products from the neoplasms.

INTRODUCTION

In the syndromes to be described, circulating agents cause intestinal secretion or changes in motility with decreased intestinal transit time, resulting in secretory-type diarrhea. Secretory diarrhea as opposed to osmotic diarrhea is characterized by large-volume, watery stools, often more than 1 L per day; by persistence of diarrhea when patients fast; and by the fact that on analysis of stool-water, measured osmolarity is identical to that calculated from the electrolytes present.[1] This calculation is done by analyzing the sodium and potassium concentrations, multiplying their sum by 2 to account for the anions, and comparing this number to the measured osmolarity.[2]

The authors have nothing to disclose.
Division of Gastroenterology and Hepatology, Department of Internal Medicine, Medical University of Graz, Graz, Austria
* Corresponding author. Division of Gastroenterology and Hepatology, Medical University of Graz, Auenbruggerplatz 15, Graz 8036, Austria.
E-mail address: guenter.krejs@medunigraz.at

Gastroenterol Clin N Am 41 (2012) 603–610
http://dx.doi.org/10.1016/j.gtc.2012.06.008
0889-8553/12/$ – see front matter © 2012 Elsevier Inc. All rights reserved.

Although sodium plays the main role in water and electrolyte absorption, chloride is the major ion involved in secretion. Several intracellular steps result in exit of chloride ions from epithelial cells through a chloride-specific channel in the apical membrane.[3] This process can be initiated from the luminal side, for instance, by cholera toxin or from the serosal side by circulating agents, such as serotonin or VIP. Both cholera toxin and VIP trigger increases in intracellular cyclic adenosine monophosphate (cAMP), which causes active chloride secretion.[4,5] A list of agents that cause secretion in vitro (applied from the serosal side of intestinal mucosa) or in vivo (as circulating agents) is given in **Table 1**.[6,7]

THE CLASSIC ENDOCRINE DIARRHEAL SYNDROME: VERNER-MORRISON SYNDROME OR VIPOMA SYNDROME

Other names for Verner-Morrison syndrome or VIPoma syndrome are pancreatic cholera syndrome and watery diarrhea hypokalemia hypochlorhydria (WDHH) syndrome. VIP is produced by a pancreatic tumor.[8] VIP under normal circumstances serves as a neurotransmitter in the peripheral and central nervous system, particularly in the enteric nervous system and in the urogenital tract. The normally seen low levels of serum VIP are viewed as a neuronal overflow phenomenon. Only in the presence of a VIP-producing tumor are the serum concentrations elevated. These tumors occur with a frequency of 1 case per 10 million population per year.

Verner and Morrison[9] of Duke University first called attention to this syndrome in association with an islet cell tumor. Before the discovery of VIP (see below) it was the hypochlorhydria that differentiated this syndrome from the Zollinger-Ellison syndrome (ZES) described 3 years previously. The name, *pancreatic cholera syndrome*, was first used by Matsumoto and coworkers.[10] Pancreatic cholera syndrome is an appropriate name because the diarrhea results from cAMP-mediated intestinal secretion, as in Asiatic cholera. The only shortcoming of this term is that some tumors are outside the pancreas (eg, ganglioneuroblastomas or other neural crest tumors). Bloom and colleagues[11] first found elevated levels of VIP in plasma and in tumor tissue of such patients.

VIP was discovered and isolated by Said and Mutt between 1968 and 1972.[12–14] It is a 28–amino acid polypeptide with a molecular weight of 3326. Initially discovered as a vasoactive substance, VIP was once viewed as a gastrointestinal hormone by Morton Grossman before it became clear that its major role is that of a neurotransmitter.

VIP is an intestinal secretagogue and causes active chloride and bicarbonate secretion by intestinal epithelia. In intestinal perfusion experiments in dogs and in humans, the authors have shown active chloride secretion (against a chemical and electrical gradient) in response to VIP.[15,16] A smaller effect can also be seen in the colon.[17] In healthy volunteers, VIP infusion over 10 hours to reach plasma levels similar to those seen in patients with pancreatic cholera can mimic the syndrome (an average of 2.4 L of stool in 10 hours).[18,19]

The large fluid loss in such patients (the authors have observed diarrhea volumes up to 10 L per day) and the loss of bicarbonate in stool water lead to metabolic acidosis

Table 1
Substances that can cause intestinal secretion

Hormones	Gastrin, secretin, cholecystokinin, glucagon, enteroglucagon, gastric inhibitory polypeptide, calcitonin
Neuroendocrine substances	Acetylcholine, VIP, peptide histidine methionine, helodermin, substance P, bombesin, neurotensin, serotonin, galanin-1, adenosine triphosphate
Other substances	Histamine, bradykinin, prostaglandins

and hypokalemia (the colon preserves sodium but loses potassium in exchange). Untreated patients die of renal failure due to hypovolemia. The authors have measured an average stool volume of 4.5 L per day in 9 such patients who were eating a regular diet (1.8 L while fasting). A typical stool collection is shown in **Fig. 1**. Resection of the tumor is the therapy of choice; however, more than 50% of the patients have liver metastases at the time of diagnosis.

Treatment with somatostatin analog has been effective[20,21] and chemotherapy with streptozotocin and 5-fluorouracil (5-FU) is also beneficial. A large armamentarium of other therapeutic options is now available, includeing targeted therapy with everolimus, radioligand therapy, and chemoembolization. In rare cases, when after resection of the primary tumor the remaining metastases are limited to the liver, partial hepatectomy or liver transplantation can be performed. In some of the tumors, other peptides are cosecreted, such as peptide histidine methionine, calcitonin, and helodermin. All these agents are capable of changing absorption to secretion in the intestine, but the main mediator of intestinal secretion and thus of diarrhea, is VIP. There is also a troublesome syndrome referred to as pseudopancreatic cholera in which no tumor or circulating secretagogue can be found in the presence of long-lasting secretory diarrhea.[22,23]

MALIGNANT CARCINOID SYNDROME

The term, *carcinoid*, goes back to the German pathologist, Siegfried Oberndorfer.[24] Carcinoid syndrome is still used to describe a clinical condition[25] but as far as morphology and histopathology are concerned these neoplasias are now classified as neuroendocrine tumors. Localized carcinoids are frequently found in the gastrointestinal tract at autopsy. The malignant carcinoid syndrome is observed practically only when metastases are present in the liver. The tumor produces serotonin, substance P, and tachykinines (neurokinin A and neuropeptide K). These agents lead to flushing, diarrhea due to intestinal secretion and fast transit, bronchospasm,

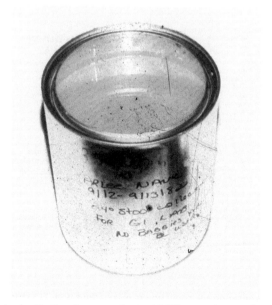

Fig. 1. A 24-hour stool collection from a patient with VIPoma. The 1-gallon (3.5-L) paint can is almost full with yellow watery stool, a pure electrolyte solution (K^+: 70 mEq/L, Na^+: 64 mEq/L).

and right-sided endocardial fibrosis. In addition to imaging studies, measurement of 24-hour urinary 5-hydroxyindoleacetic acid (5-HIAA) is most important for diagnosis. With multiple liver metastases, 24-hour urinary 5-HIAA excretion is often in the range of 70 mg to 250 mg. As for neuroendocrine tumors in general, chromogranin A in serum is also a good marker for tumor mass and prognosis.[26] Because the primary tumor is often in the ileum and may lead to small-bowel obstruction (due to the tumor itself or to retractile mesenteritis), surgical resection is necessary. It is not infrequent that small bowel obstruction is the presenting symptom. The positive aspect of this presentation is early resection of the primary tumor, however, complete resection of all tumor is often not accomplished during emergency surgery. For metastases in the liver, chemoembolization may often be successful. Treatment with somatostatin analogs is broadly applied.[27,28] Addition of interferon and cytotoxic chemotherapy is another option. Management guidelines for neuroendocrine tumor are now available from the European Neuroendocrine Tumor Society.[29,30] Because rapid transit plays an important role, antimotility drugs (loperamide and codeine phosphate) may alone markedly improve the diarrhea.

ZOLLINGER-ELLISON SYNDROME

In ZES,[31] gastrin-producing tumors cause acid hypersecretion and the hallmark is severe peptic ulcer disease, usually with complications, such as bleeding and perforation. Approximately 10% of patients, however, present with watery diarrhea as the first and sometimes disabling symptom. Diarrhea per se is present in approximately 50% to 60% of patients who have untreated ZES. Here, the mechanism of diarrhea is different from other secretory diarrheas. It is the increased gastric secretion with large fluid volumes that enter the small bowel that overwhelms the absorptive capacity of the intestine . Diarrheal volume is often in excess of 1 L per day. In one patient whom the authors have studied by siphonage and perfusion techniques, the transit volume in the upper jejunum amounted to approximately 15 L in 24 hours while fasting (**Fig. 2**). In

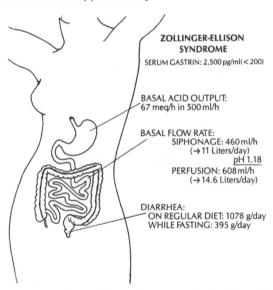

ZOLLINGER-ELLISON
SYNDROME
SERUM GASTRIN: 2,500 pg/ml (< 200)

BASAL ACID OUTPUT:
67 meq/h in 500 ml/h

BASAL FLOW RATE:
SIPHONAGE: 460 ml/h
(→ 11 Liters/day)
pH 1.18
PERFUSION: 608 ml/h
(→ 14.6 Liters/day)

DIARRHEA:
ON REGULAR DIET: 1078 g/day
WHILE FASTING: 395 g/day

Fig. 2. Flow volumes entering the small bowel in a patient with ZES studied by the authors. A large dose of the H₂-blocker, cimetidine, reduced the diarrhea markedly. After the gastrinoma was surgically removed, diarrhea stopped completely.

some patients, volumes up to 23 L have been observed.[32] The diarrhea disappears after acid secretion has been controlled by proton pump inhibitors.

Mild steatorrhea is also present in such patients (eg, 12 g of stool fat per day [normal is up to 7]) and this is due to the inactivation of lipase in the small bowel by the low luminal pH. Circulating gastrin may also have an antiabsorptive effect.[33] Treatment is aimed at controlling acid secretion and attempting to remove the tumor. ZES is now diagnosed earlier due to the availability of the intravenous secretin test, despite modern imaging techniques finding the primary tumor may still be difficult. In advanced cases, treatment aims at controlling of tumor mass with cytotoxic agents. Also, approximately 25% of gastrinomas occur in the setting of multiple endocrine neoplasia type 1 and need special management.[34,35]

MEDULLARY CARCINOMA OF THE THYROID

Diarrhea occurs in 30% of patients with medullary carcinoma of the thyroid and may precede the presence of a palpable thyroid mass. In human intestinal perfusion experiments, calcitonin has been shown to change water and electrolyte movement from absorption to secretion.[36] Circulating calcitonin is the major mediator of intestinal secretion in this syndrome. A motility factor with decreased transit time may also play a role (diarrhée motrice [motor diarrhea]).[37] Because this tumor may be part of multiple endocrine neoplasia types 2 and 3, first-degree relatives need to be genetically screened for the mutation or investigated by measuring basal and post-provocation (intravenous pentagastrin) plasma calcitonin concentration. Other than in medullary carcinoma of the thyroid, calcitonin is found in high concentrations in plasma and tumor tissue of several patients with endocrine pancreatic tumors (VIPoma or somatistatinoma) but only in rare instances is it the single or predominant polypeptide.[38,39]

SOMATOSTATINOMA SYNDROME

Somatostatinoma syndrome is a rare tumor syndrome first described by the authors.[40] It is estimated to occur in approximately 1 in 40 million population per year. Somatostatin inhibits most functions in the digestive tract.[41] It causes steatorrhea due to inhibition of pancreatic secretion and this is the main cause of diarrhea in such patients. Whether a shortened interval between migrating myoelectric complexes[40] plays a role in the cause of this diarrhea is not clear. Some patients have cosecretion of calcitonin, which can act as intestinal secretagogue. Therapy consists of tumor resection and chemotherapy (streptozotocin and 5-FU).

SYSTEMIC MASTOCYTOSIS

Increased release of histamine from mast cells has several effects on the gastrointestinal tract. It increases gastric acid secretion and shifts water and electrolyte absorption from absorption to secretion and may have a prokinetic effect. Steatorrhea may also be present.[42] Diarrhea and other symptoms (including flush) are often episodic.[37,42]

HYPERTHYROIDISM

The mechanisms of diarrhea in hyperthyroidism have not been studied extensively, because therapy is begun promptly after the diagnosis is established in such patients. Diarrhea is present in 10% to 40% of patients and is episodic. Decreased intestinal transit time is believed to be the main cause.[37]

OTHER CAUSES

Diarrhea has been reported in tumors producing pancreatic polypeptide (PP).[43] PP itself may serve as a marker of pancreatic endocrine tumors.[44] Diarrhea may occur in 1 of 5 patients with the glucagonoma syndrome, where migratory necrolytic erythema is a hallmark (the incidence of glucagonoma is only 1 in 20 million population per year).[45] There are no unequivocal reports of secretinomas, a tumor containing and releasing the poypeptide for which the term, *hormone*, was first coined in 1902.[46] The authors have studied a child with life-threatening diarrhea and apparent VIPoma but helodermin was more prominent in plasma than VIP.

REFERENCES

1. Krejs GJ. Diarrhea. In: Wyngaarden JB, Smith LH, editors. Cecil. Textbook of medicine. 19th edition. Philadelphia: W.B. Saunders; 1992. p. 680–7.
2. Krejs GJ, Hendler RS, Fordtran JS. Diagnostic and pathophysiologic studies in patients with chronic diarrhea. In: Field M, editor. Secretory diarrhea. Bethesda (MD): American Physiological Society; 1980. p. 141–51.
3. Bridges RJ, Rummel W. Mechanistic basis of alterations in mucosal water and electrolyte transport. Clin Gastroenterol 1986;15:491–506.
4. Field M. Regulation of small intestinal ion transport by cyclic nucleotides and calcium. In: Field M, editor. Secretory diarrhea. Bethesda (MD): American Physiological Society; 1980. p. 21–30.
5. Field M. Intestinal ion transport and the pathophysiology of diarrhea. J Clin Invest 2003;111:931–43.
6. Krejs GJ. Secretory diarrhea. Triangle 1988;27:143–8.
7. Jones SL, Blikslager AT. Role of the enteric nervous system in the pathophysiology of secretory diarrhea. J Vet Intern Med 2002;16:222–8.
8. Krejs GJ. VIPoma Syndrome. Am J Gastroenterol 1987;82:38–48.
9. Verner JV, Morrison AB. Islet cell tumor and a syndrome of refractory watery diarrhea and hypokalemia. Am J Med 1958;25:374–80.
10. Matsumoto KK, Peter JB, Schultze RG, et al. Watery diarrhea and hypokalemia associated with pancreatic islet cell adenoma. Gastroenterology 1966;50: 231–42.
11. Bloom SR, Polak JM, Pearse AGE. Vasoactive intestinal peptide and watery-diarrrhea syndrome. Lancet 1973;2:14–6.
12. Said SI, Mutt V. Potent peripheral and splanchnic vasodilator peptide from normal gut. Nature 1970;225:863–4.
13. Said SI, Mutt V. Polypeptide with broad biological activity: isolation from small intestine. Science 1970;169:1217–8.
14. Said SI, Mutt V. Isolation from porcine intestinal wall of a vasoactive octacosapeptide related to secretin and glucagon. Eur J Biochem 1972;28:199–204.
15. Krejs GJ, Barkley RM, Read NW, et al. Intestinal secretion induced by vasoactive intestinal polypeptide. A comparison with choleratoxin in the canine jejunum in vivo. J Clin Invest 1978;61:1337–45.
16. Krejs GJ, Fordtran JS, Bloom SR, et al. Effect of VIP infusion on water and ion transport in the human jejunum. Gastroenterology 1980;78:722–7.
17. Krejs GJ. Effect of VIP infusion on water and electrolyte transport in the human intestine. In: Said SI, editor. Vasoactive intestinal peptide. New York: Raven Press; 1982. p. 193–200.
18. Kane MG, O'Dorisio TM, Krejs GJ. Intravenous VIP infusion causes secretory diarrhea in man. N Engl J Med 1983;309:1482–5.

19. Krejs GJ, Kane MG, O'Dorisio TM. VIP and the pancreatic cholera syndrome. N Engl J Med 1984;310:1465–6.
20. Santangelo WC, O'Dorisio TM, Kim JG, et al. Effect of synthetic somatostatin analogue on intestinal water and ion transport in pancreatic cholera syndrome. Ann Intern Med 1985;103:364–7.
21. Santangelo WC, O'Dorisio TM, Kim JG, et al. VIPoma syndrome: effect of a synthetic somatostatin analogue. Scand J Gastroenterol 1986;21(Suppl 119): 87–90.
22. Read NW, Read MG, Krejs GJ, et al. A report of five patients with large-volume secretory diarrhea but no evidence of endocrine tumor or laxative abuse. Dig Dis Sci 1982;27:193–201.
23. Santangelo WC, Dueno MI, Krejs GJ. Pseudopancreatic cholera. Effect of a synthetic somatostatin analogue. Am J Med 1987;82(Suppl 5B):84–7.
24. Oberndorfer S. Karzinoide Tumore des Duenndarms. Frankf Z Pathol 1907;1: 426–32.
25. Modlin IM, Lye KD, Kidd M. A 5-decade analysis of 13,715 carcinoid tumors. Cancer 2003;97:934–59.
26. Arnold R, Wilke A, Rinke A, et al. Plasma chromogranin A as marker for survival in patients with metastatic endocrine gastroenteropancreatic tumors. Clin Gastroenterol Hepatol 2008;6:820–7.
27. Davis GR, Camp RC, Raskin P, et al. Effect of somatostatin infusion on jejunal water and electrolyte transport in a patient with secretory diarrhea due to malignant carcinoid syndrome. Gastroenterology 1980;78:346–9.
28. Modlin IM, Pavel M, Kidd M, et al. Review article: somatostatin analogues in the treatment of gastroenteropancreatic neuroendocrine (carcinoid) tumors. Aliment Pharmacol Ther 2010;31:169–88.
29. ENETS Consensus Guidelines for the Management of Patients with Digestive Neuroendocrine Tumors Part 1—Stomach, Duodenum and Pancreas. Neuroendocrinology 2006;84:151–216.
30. ENETS Consensus Guidelines for the Management of Patients with Digestive Neuroendocrine Tumors Part 2—Midgut and Hindgut Tumors. Neuroendocrinology 2008;87:1–64.
31. Zollinger RM, Ellison EH. Primary peptic ulceracion of the jejunum associated with islet cell tumors of the pancreas. Ann Surg 1955;142:709–28.
32. Rambaud JC, Modigliani R, Emonts P, et al. Fluid secretion in the duodenum and intestinal handling of water and electrolytes in Zollinger-Ellision syndrome. Dig Dis 1978;23:1089–97.
33. Wright HK, Hersh T, Floch MH, et al. Impaired absorption in the Zollinger-Ellison syndrome independent of gastric hypersecretion. Am J Surg 1970;119:250–3.
34. Jensen RT. Pancreatic endocrine tumors: recent advances. Ann Oncol 1999; 10(Suppl 4):S170–6.
35. Warner RR. Enteroendocrine tumors other than carcinoid: a review of clinically significant advances. Gastroenterology 2005;128:1668–84.
36. Gray IK, Brannan P, Juan D, et al. Ion transport changes during calcitonin-induced intestinal secretion in man. Gastroenterology 1976;71:392–8.
37. Rambaud JC, Hautefeuille M, Ruskone A, et al. Diarrhea due to circulating agents. Clin Gastroenterol 1986;15:603–29.
38. Mullerpatan PM, Joshi SR, Shah RC, et al. Calcitonin-secreting tumor of the pancreas. Dig Surg 2004;21:321–4.
39. Jarufe NP, Coldham C, Orug T, et al. Neuroendocrine tumors of the pancreas: predictors of survival after surgical treatment. Dig Surg 2005;22:157–62.

40. Krejs GJ, Orci L, Conlon JM, et al. Somatostatinoma syndrome: biochemical, morphologic and clinical features. N Engl J Med 1979;301:285–92.

41. Krejs GJ, Browne R, Raskin P. Effect of intravenous somatostatin on jejunal absorption of glucose, amino acids, water and electrolytes. Gastroenterology 1980;78:26–31.

42. Bredfeldt JE, O'Laughlin JC, Burham JB, et al. Malabsorption and gastric hypersecretion in systemic mastocytosis. Am J Gastroenterol 1980;74:133–7.

43. Lundqvist G, Krause U, Larsson LI, et al. A pancreatic-polypeptide-producing tumor associated with the WDHA Syndrome. Scand J Gastroenterol 1978;13:715–8.

44. Adrian TE, Uttenthal LO, Williams SJ, et al. Secretion of pancreatic polypeptide in patients with pancreatic endocrine tumors. N Engl J Med 1986;315:287–91.

45. van Beek AP, de Haas ER, van Vloten WA. The gulcagonoma syndrome and necrolytic migratory erythema: a clinical review. Eur J Endocrinol 2004;151:531–7.

46. Bayliss WM, Starling E. The mechanism of pancreatic secretion. J Physiol 1902;28:325–53.

Diarrhea Caused By Carbohydrate Malabsorption

Heinz F. Hammer, MD[a,b,*], Johann Hammer, MD[c]

KEYWORDS

- Lactose • Fructose • Antibiotics • Colonic transit • Dietary fiber • Intestinal gas

KEY POINTS

- Diarrhea in carbohydrate malabsorption is due to acceleration of colonic transit and the osmotic load of carbohydrates, short chain fatty acids, and electrolytes.
- Short chain fatty acids inhibit colonic transit, and their effect on transit deserves further evaluation for a possible clinical role in slow-transit constipation.
- Diarrhea associated with antibiotics may result from inhibition of colonic salvage of incompletely absorbed carbohydrates.
- In patients with lactose malabsorption, the association between malabsorption and abdominal symptoms has to be established.
- If lactose intolerance symptoms persist on a lactose restricted diet, other substrates for colonic bacterial metabolism, like dietary fibers or fructose, have to be restricted as well.

INTRODUCTION

The term carbohydrate malabsorption is used to describe conditions in which carbo-hydrates escape digestion and/or absorption in the small intestine and reach the colon. Although this is usually considered to be a consequence of a malabsorptive disease of the pancreas or small intestine, carbohydrates also reach the colon in phys-iologically incomplete carbohydrate absorption. This is due to ingestion of carbohy-drates for which the healthy gastrointestinal (GI) tract of the human has a limited digestive or absorptive capacity. Carbohydrate malabsorption may result in symp-toms due to complete or incomplete bacterial metabolism of carbohydrates in the colon. These symptoms are bloating, abdominal cramping, passing of gas, flatulence,

The authors have nothing to disclose.

This work was supported by research grants P 18101-B09 and L309-B09 from the Austrian Science Fund (FWF, Fonds zur Förderung der wissenschaftlichen Forschung) to Dr J. Hammer.

[a] Division of Gastroenterology and Hepatology, Department of Internal Medicine, Medical University of Graz, Auenbruggerplatz 15, Graz 8036, Austria; [b] Privatklinik Kastanienhof, Grit-zenweg 16, Graz 8052, Austria; [c] Division of Gastroenterology and Hepatology, Department of Internal Medicine, Medical University of Vienna, Währinger Gürtel 18–20, Vienna 1090, Austria
* Corresponding author. Division of Gastroenterology and Hepatology, Department of Internal Medicine, Medical University of Graz, Auenbruggerplatz 15, Graz 8036, Austria.
E-mail address: heinz.hammer@medunigraz.at

Gastroenterol Clin N Am 41 (2012) 611–627
http://dx.doi.org/10.1016/j.gtc.2012.06.003
0889-8553/12/$ – see front matter © 2012 Elsevier Inc. All rights reserved.

and diarrhea (carbohydrate intolerance). It is important for physicians and for patients to remember that carbohydrate intolerance does not necessarily imply that a malabsorptive disease is present, but may be the result of individual dietary habits or intolerances, probably related to increased intestinal sensitivities.

Symptoms of carbohydrate intolerance may result from

1. Inborn or acquired defects of luminal or membrane bound pancreatic or intestinal enzymes that are needed for digestion of polysaccharides, oligosaccharides, or disaccharides
2. Decreased absorption of monosaccharides due to primary defects in mucosal absorptive mechanisms or secondary to extensive reduction of small intestinal absorptive surface area due to small bowel diseases or extensive resections
3. Ingesting carbohydrates for which there is a physiologically limited or totally absent digestive and/or absorptive capacity, like fructose, mannitol, sorbitol, or dietary fibers
4. Adverse effects of therapy or dietary intervention with nonabsorbable carbohydrates (lactulose, lactitol), drugs interfering with carbohydrate absorption (acarbose, metformin), or sugar exchange products (sorbitol, fructose)
5. Antibiotics interfering with colonic salvage of malabsorbed or physiologically incompletely absorbed carbohydrates

This article will focus on the role of the colon in the pathogenesis of diarrhea in carbohydrate malabsorption or physiologically incomplete absorption of carbohydrates, and on the most common manifestation of carbohydrate malabsorption, lactose malabsorption. In addition, incomplete fructose absorption, the role of carbohydrate malabsorption in other malabsorptive diseases, and congenital defects that lead to malabsorption will be covered. The article concludes with a section on diagnostic tools to evaluate carbohydrate malabsorption.

METHODS FOR ESTABLISHING THE ROLE OF CARBOHYDRATE MALABSORPTION FOR THE PATHOGENESIS OF DIARRHEA

Carbohydrates that are not absorbed in the small intestine are metabolized by colonic bacteria to organic acids. These organic acids are lactic acid and the short chain fatty acids respectively their salts acetate, propionate and butyrate. Most of the organic acids are absorbed across the colonic mucosa.[1,2] Carbohydrates that are not metabolized by colonic bacteria to organic acids, and organic acids that escape absorption by the colon, remain in the colonic lumen and lead to osmotic diarrhea and fecal calorie loss.[3,4]

Whether carbohydrates exert osmotic activity in the colon, thereby resulting in colonic water and electrolyte accumulation and diarrhea, depends on their molar concentration (expressed in mmol/L). For assessment of their osmotic activity, products of bacterial carbohydrate metabolism, that is organic acids, have to be taken into account. Lastly, for calculation of the osmotic activity of malabsorbed or incompletely absorbed carbohydrates, also the cations, which are bound by anionic salts of organic acids, have to be considered. The authors have previously established that 1 mmol of fecal organic acids obligates an average of 0.6 mmol cations (0.30 mmol Na, 0.21 mmol Ca, 0.07 mmol K, and 0.02 mmol Mg).[3,4]

A comprehensive picture of the magnitude of carbohydrate malabsorption and its significance for the pathogenesis of diarrhea in malabsorptive diseases was gained in studies in which fecal outputs of carbohydrates and organic acids were measured in normal subjects with diarrhea induced by ingestion of lactulose, and in patients with severe malabsorption.[3,4] Carbohydrates were assayed in 24-hour stool collections using anthrone, a method that measures all hexose carbohydrates, whether excreted as monosaccharides, disaccharides, or oligosaccharides.[3–6] The unit of expression is grams excreted per day. This method provided a measure of total fecal carbohydrate excretion, regardless of molecular size. A reducing sugar assay[3,7] was used to detect the reducing ends of carbohydrate molecules; 1 mol of starch (>50,000 g of carbohydrate) and 1 mol of glucose (180 g of carbohydrate) give the same result. Therefore, the reducing sugar assay provided information on the number of moles of excreted carbohydrate and was used to determine the osmotic effect of fecal carbohydrates. The reducing sugar assay has to be performed in lyophilized stool samples that have been reconstituted to their original weight by adding water to remove noncarbohydrate volatile reducing substances.[3] In a later study, individual carbohydrates were measured by high-performance liquid chromatography (HPLC), and their molar or gram amounts were calculated by summing individual carbohydrates.[8–11]

Fecal output of total organic acids quantifies the fraction of carbohydrates that are excreted in stool as a bacterial product of unabsorbed carbohydrates. In initial studies analyzing their osmotic effects and outputs[3,4] organic acids were analyzed by titration assay, which measures total organic acid concentration[4,12]; in a later study by the authors' group, individual acids were measured by HPLC.[8–11]

In summary, to assess osmotic activity and the role of carbohydrate malabsorption for the pathogenesis of diarrhea, the sum of carbohydrates plus organic acids plus cations (that is measured organic acids in mmol/L $\times$ 0.6) has to be calculated and expressed as millimoles per liter. In diarrhea with only slightly increased stool weight, organic acids and electrolytes are the main driving force of carbohydrate-induced osmotic diarrhea. Only in severe carbohydrate malabsorption, with stool weight in excess of 500 g/d fecal, does carbohydrate excretion become a driving force.

THE ROLE OF THE COLON FOR COLONIC SALVAGE OF MALABSORBED OR INCOMPLETELY ABSORBED CARBOHYDRATES AND GAS PRODUCTION

The colon has the capacity to absorb a limited variety of nutrients and minerals. Although colonic nutrient absorption does not play a major role in health, the nutritive role of the colon in patients with severe malabsorption has been demonstrated.[13]

In healthy people, between 2% and 20% of ingested starch escapes absorption in the small intestine[14]; pancreatic insufficiency and severe intestinal disorders further increase this amount.[3] Carbohydrates that reach the colon cannot be absorbed by the colonic mucosa but can be metabolized by the bacterial flora. Anaerobic bacterial metabolism results in the breakdown of oligosaccharides and polysaccharides to mono- and disaccharides, which are metabolized further to lactic acid and short-chain (C2 to C4) fatty acids, such as acetate, propionate, and butyrate, and to odorless gases, including hydrogen, methane, and carbon dioxide.[15] Although considerable proportions of these organic acids and gases are absorbed by the colonic mucosa,[2,16] some remain in the colon, resulting in diarrhea[3,4] and symptoms due to gas-like bloating, flatulence, and cramping.[17,18] The same principle also applies to dietary fibers, which have been calculated to contain 2.5 to 3.1 kcal of metabolizable energy per gram fiber, which is liberated and made available for colonic absorption.[19]

Studies in normal subjects have shown that the bacterial metabolism of starch to small carbohydrate moieties is a rapid process in the normal colon. The rate-limiting step in the overall conversion of polysaccharides to short-chain fatty acids is the conversion of monosaccharides to short-chain fatty acids.[3] Colonic absorption of short-chain fatty acids[2] results in a reduction of the osmotic load and in mitigation of diarrhea. In normal subjects, more than 45 g of carbohydrates must reach the colon to cause diarrhea, and up to 80 g of carbohydrates per day can be metabolized by bacteria to short-chain fatty acids; approximately 90% of these short-chain fatty acids are absorbed by colonic mucosa.[4] Chronic carbohydrate malabsorption causes adaptive changes in bacterial metabolic activity that result in an even higher efficiency of the bacterial flora to digest carbohydrates[20] although at the expense of increased flatus production.

Because short-chain fatty acids have caloric values between 3.4 and 5.95 kcal/g,[21] colonic absorption of these acids decreases caloric loss in carbohydrate malabsorption. In patients with short bowel syndrome, colonic salvage of malabsorbed carbohydrates can contribute up to 700– to 950 kcal/d, provided that a substantial part of the colon remains in continuity with the small bowel.[22]

The beneficial effects of colonic bacterial carbohydrate metabolism are accompanied by side effects due to gas production. Up to 8-fold interindividual differences in the volume of gas produced in the colon have been observed in normal persons after a dose of 12.5 g lactulose[16,18] The colon can absorb gas; if intracolonic gas volumes are low, up to 90% of the volume of intracolonic gas can be absorbed. However, if gas volumes are high, this proportion decreases to as low as 20%.[16] Therefore, persons who have the disadvantage of producing more gas in their colon have an additional disadvantage in that they absorb a smaller fraction of the gas. Gas produced from bacterial carbohydrate metabolism is odorless. The odor of flatus is due to volatile sulfur-containing substrates that result from bacterial metabolism of protein.[23]

Impaired colonic salvage of carbohydrates has been suggested to contribute to the diarrhea in Crohn disease[24] and ulcerative colitis.[25] Bacterial carbohydrate metabolism may be decreased by antibiotic treatment.[26] In some patients, antibiotic-associated diarrhea may be the result of impaired colonic salvage of physiologically incompletely absorbed carbohydrates or dietary fibers, which may accumulate in stool because of decreased bacterial fermentation.[27]

INFLUENCE OF ANTIBIOTICS ON COLONIC CARBOHYDRATE SALVAGE

It has been suggested that in normal subjects, as much as 70 g of carbohydrates reaches the colon per day.[14,17] The colon cannot absorb carbohydrates, but colonic bacteria metabolize carbohydrates as an energy source, thereby reducing osmotic load and salvaging calories for the human host.

Inhibition of bacterial carbohydrate metabolism by antibiotics may result in an increase of osmotically active solutes in the colon, resulting in osmotic diarrhea. In addition, reduced production of organic acids may result in functional disturbances of colonic mucosa. In the distal colon, the short chain fatty acid (SCFA) n-butyrate is an important source of energy for the mucosa through cellular oxidation.[28,29] Reduction in SCFA production may deprive the colonic mucosa of an energy source, as demonstrated by the clinical model of exclusion colitis (diversion colitis) in patients with exclusion of distal parts of the colon from the fecal stream.[30]

Various antibiotics have been shown to reduce colonic bacterial carbohydrate metabolism.[27,31–35] Reduction of carbohydrate metabolism can result in osmotic diarrhea. However, the development of diarrhea is dependent on the quantity of poorly absorbable dietary carbohydrates like vegetables and dietary fibers.[32,34]

An in vitro study simulating luminal contents of the proximal colon has demonstrated that clindamycin reduces anaerobes (clostridium and bacteroides species), decreases fecal carbohydrate metabolism, and decreases concentrations of SCFA.[31] Ampicillin reduces colonic bacterial carbohydrate fermentation, as shown by a decreased breath hydrogen response and by the presence of carbohydrates in stool.[32]

Inhibition of carbohydrate salvage contributes to the development of diarrhea, as indicated by an increase in frequency and stool weight in subjects who ingested a subdiarrheal dose of lactulose.[32,33] Reduced colonic carbohydrate fermentation has also been shown to occur in healthy subjects following oral administration of ampicillin and metronidazole.[27,34] Patients with diarrhea associated with pivampicillin, dicloxacillin, erythromycin, or ampicillin plus netilmicin had reduced fecal concentrations of SCFA. In the same study, another group of patients treated with erythromycin, dicloxacillin, or a combination of ampicillin, netilmicin, and metronidazole also had reduced fecal concentrations of SCFA but did not develop diarrhea. However, monotherapy with penicillin or pivampicillin did not reduce fecal SCFA concentrations or result in diarrhea.[35]

In another study, SCFA concentrations were measured in the stool of 15 liver-transplanted patients who received bowel-suppressing antibiotics consisting of cefuroxime, tobramycin, and nystatin. Thirteen of them developed *Clostridium difficile*-negative diarrhea, and the levels of SCFA in the stools were very low, possibly because of nearly complete suppression of colonic bacterial fermentation. The diarrhea resolved before cessation of antibiotic therapy and normalization of the fecal SCFA levels.[36]

Although fecal carbohydrates were measured in none of these studies, decreased SCFA concentrations most likely indicate decreased bacterial metabolism of incompletely absorbed carbohydrates.

Discrepancies between suppression of carbohydrate metabolism and manifestation of diarrhea[35,36] suggest that disturbed carbohydrate metabolism was not the only mechanism responsible for diarrhea. A possible reason for the observed discrepancies may be an adaptive increase in colonic transit time. It has been shown that colonic transit time in osmotic diarrhea increases in the descending colon.[37] This may provide more time for metabolism of carbohydrates and absorption of SCFA, water, and electrolytes.

THE ROLE OF COLONIC TRANSIT IN CARBOHYDRATE-INDUCED DIARRHEA

Diarrhea that develops due to malabsorbed carbohydrates may be seen as the failure of colonic salvage. This may be due to excessive amounts of carbohydrate entering the colon, or decreased time available for metabolism of malabsorbed carbohydrates and absorption of organic acids and electrolytes. Accelerated colonic transit (that is decreased transit time) may result from an increase in the volume load to the colon, a change in the composition of the substrate entering the colon, or an alteration of colonic motility. Accelerated transit decreases time available for storage, bacterial metabolism, and absorption.

Malabsorption of carbohydrates in the small intestine can increase the volume that flows from the ileum into the colon to as much as 10 L/d.[38] While an increase of the colonic fluid load per se accelerates colonic transit, especially transit through the proximal colon,[39] the colon also possesses an ability to accommodate and store excess fluid volumes.[37] When the storage capacity of the proximal colon is surpassed, the distal colon may provide reserve capacity that may provide additional time to absorb and metabolize colonic contents.[37] The total time the colonic contents reside in the lumen is important for providing the time for bacterial metabolism of carbohydrates and for mucosal absorption of organic acids, electrolytes, and fluids. Under optimal conditions, the colon can absorb as much as 6 L of electrolyte solutions.[40] However, the osmotic forces in carbohydrate malabsorption counteract the absorptive capacity of the colonic mucosa.[3,4] Carbohydrate malabsorption results in a dose-dependent acceleration of colonic transit[11,41] as a result of a fluid overload of the colon.

A study that compared the effect of malabsorbed degradable carbohydrates (lactulose) on colonic transit with an osmotically active, nondegradable solution (polyethylene glycol, PEG) demonstrated that carbohydrate malabsorption has a differential effect on colonic transit.[11] An acceleration of colonic transit during carbohydrate ingestion takes place secondary to an increased intracolonic volume. This is partly counteracted by slowing of transit due to short chain fatty acids. The high concentration of short chain fatty acids in carbohydrate malabsorption reduces colonic motor activity.[42] In the study comparing colonic transit in lactulose and PEG-induced diarrhea, increased short chain fatty acid concentrations resulted in an inhibition of colonic transit as compared with similar osmotic loads of PEG.[11]

The size of the differences in colonic transit during ingestion of lactulose and PEG at doses that result in similar severity of diarrhea, as assessed by 24-hour stool weight, is quite remarkable; during ingestion of lactulose, there is a delay in mean residence time of colonic contents in the distal colon by 250% as compared with PEG ingestion. Mean residence time in the total colon after lactulose is also increased, but only by 50% as compared with PEG.[11] Therefore due to the composition of colonic contents during carbohydrate malabsorption, the colon can accommodate up to 6 times higher osmotic loads of malabsorbed carbohydrates as compared with osmotic loads of PEG.

The complex relation between colonic contents, colonic volume, and transit during carbohydrate malabsorption provides further explanation for the nonlinear dose–effect curve of lactulose,[4] in that bacterial metabolism of lactulose and absorption of its metabolic products (that is organic acids) do not only result in a reduction of the osmotic load, but also have slowing effects on colonic transit, which in turn may result in increased time for bacterial metabolism of carbohydrates and mucosal absorption of short chain fatty acids.

The inhibitory effects of short chain fatty acids on colonic transit deserve further evaluation for their possible clinical role in the pathogenesis and treatment of slow transit constipation. Short chain fatty acids are products of bacterial metabolism of dietary fibers, which, because of their bulking effect and the presumed acceleration of colonic transit,[43] are a first-line treatment of constipation. Treatment failure of dietary fibers could be related to inhibitory effects of short chain fatty acids on transit in some susceptible patients.

DIARRHEA IN CARBOHYDRATE MALABSORPTION—MULTIPLE INFLUENCING FACTORS

Several effects influence the clinical manifestation of diarrhea in carbohydrate malabsorption. First, osmotic fluid retention due to carbohydrates, organic acids, and electrolytes results in a dose-dependent acceleration of colonic transit, primarily in the proximal but also in the distal colon. Second, stool weight in carbohydrate malabsorption is correlated to colonic transit, but it is primarily influenced by the unabsorbed osmotic load of carbohydrates, short chain fatty acids, and electrolytes. Third, stool consistency is influenced both by stool composition (carbohydrates, organic acids, electrolytes) and transit in the distal colon. Fourth, at similar stool weight, colonic transit is significantly slower during carbohydrate malabsorption as compared with colonic volume load of other origins.[11]

CARBOHYDRATE MALABSORPTION IN MALABSORPTIVE DISEASES: INNOCENT BYSTANDER OR RELEVANT FOR CALORIE LOSS AND DIARRHEA?

In an analysis of 19 patients with severe malabsorption syndrome, 12 patients had excessive fecal excretion of carbohydrates and organic acids. In 6 of these 19 patients, carbohydrate malabsorption was a major cause of diarrhea. Furthermore, carbohydrate malabsorption contributed significantly to fecal calorie loss in some of these patients.[3]

Patients with combined small bowel and colon resection had abnormally high fecal excretion of carbohydrates and organic acids (between 11 and 78 g/d, normal being up to 5 g/d). Two factors probably contributed to high fecal excretion of carbohydrates and organic acids after small bowel plus colon resection. First, the shortened small intestine of these subjects might absorb an abnormally small fraction of ingested dietary carbohydrates, and second, their colonic conversion of carbohydrates to organic acids and their colonic absorption of these acids might be reduced.

Three of 5 patients with pancreatic disease also had excessive fecal excretion of carbohydrates and organic acids (9–21 g/d), but in these cases excess fecal carbohydrate excretion was relatively mild compared with fecal fat excretion, which was between 30 and 113 g/d in these patients.

Two of 6 patients with villous atrophy had excessive fecal excretion of carbohydrates and organic acids (14 and 103 g/d, respectively), and 1 patient had the highest fecal carbohydrate excretion of the entire group.

In 2 patients, fecal calories due to carbohydrates and organic acids approached fecal calories due to fat.

In 3 of the 5 patients with pancreatic diseases values for osmotically active reducing sugars plus organic acids plus obligated cations suggested, diarrhea was mainly due to the osmotic activity of malabsorbed carbohydrates. In 2 of those 3 patients, organic acids were excreted in excessive amounts more often than osmotically active carbohydrates of small molecular size. Also in 2 of the patients with intestinal resection and in 1 of the patients with villous atrophy, carbohydrate malabsorption was the dominant mediator of increased fecal water output.

In the other 13 patients with malabsorption syndrome, the data do not suggest a major role for carbohydrate malabsorption as a mediator of increased fecal water output even though several of them had increased fecal output of carbohydrates, however not in an osmotically relevant form.[3] This means that carbohydrates were in a large molecular form (eg, starch).

DOES CARBOHYDRATE MALABSORPTION CONTRIBUTE TO FECAL ENERGY LOSS IN ROUX-EN-Y GASTRIC BYPASS?

The long-limb Roux-en-Y gastric bypass (RYGB) has become a widely used operation for morbid obesity. In an extensive metabolic study on 9 severely obese patients before and up to 14 months after an RYGB, this operation had no significant effect on stool weight, fecal water content, or bowel movement frequency.[44] Carbohydrates comprised almost 50% of the dietary intake of combustible energy in these patients, both before and after bypass. Before bypass, coefficients of carbohydrate absorption (defined as net absorption divided by dietary intake, multiplied by 100 to derive a percentage) averaged 98%. Long-limb RYGB did not reduce the carbohydrate absorption coefficients, although carbohydrate intake was markedly reduced after RYGB.[44] The authors suggested several factors that may account for the minimal effect of long-limb RYGB on carbohydrate malabsorption. After bypass, more than one-third of dietary carbohydrate intake was composed of sugars, which should be well digested and absorbed in the Roux limb by mucosal disaccharidases and sodium–glucose cotransport. Starch can be digested by salivary amylase in the mouth and gastric pouch, and the digestive products could then be absorbed in the Roux limb. Further carbohydrate digestion and absorption occurs in the common channel, which contains the relatively indestructible pancreatic amylase.[45] If any carbohydrate escapes absorption in the small intestine, colonic bacteria would convert it to short chain fatty acids, a substantial fraction of which would be absorbed by colonic mucosa.[4]

LACTASE DEFICIENCY AND LACTOSE MALABSORPTION

Deficiency of the intestinal brush border enzyme lactase may lead to lactose malabsorption, which may result in lactose intolerance. Several causes for lactase deficiency in infants and adults have been recognized.

Unlike other intestinal disaccharidases, which develop early in fetal life, lactase levels remain low until the 34th week of gestation.[46] Transient lactase deficiency in premature infants may lead to symptoms of lactose malabsorption, such as diarrhea, until normal intestinal lactase activity develops.

In rare cases, enzyme deficiency is manifested at the time of birth and is permanent (congenital lactase deficiency).[47]

Secondary lactase deficiency may occur as a consequence of extensive small bowel diseases, like celiac disease, or extensive small bowel resections.[48] Reversible lactase deficiency may occur at all ages as a result of transient small bowel injury associated with acute diarrheal illnesses.

Acquired primary lactase deficiency (adult-type hypolactasia) is the most common form of lactase deficiency worldwide. Most populations lose considerable lactase activity in adulthood.[49] The decline in lactase activity begins soon after weaning[50] and is a multifactorial process that is regulated at the gene transcription level[51] and leads to decreased biosynthesis or retardation of intracellular transport or maturation of the enzyme lactase–phlorizin hydrolase. In white persons, a single-nucleotide polymorphism (SNP) -13910 T/C upstream of the gene coding for the enzyme lactase–phlorizin hydrolase (LPH gene) has been found to be involved in the regulation of lactase–phlorizin hydrolase.[52,53] In Europeans and their descendants, the CC genotype of the SNP -13910 T/C upstream of the LPH gene is associated with adult-type hypolactasia; TC and TT genotypes are linked with lactase persistence.[54] This polymorphism can be used as a diagnostic test for adult-type hypolactasia.[55] Other SNPs are linked to adult-type hypolactasia in Africans.[56]

Since acquired primary lactase deficiency is present in the majority of the adult human population, it has to be considered as normal, rather than as an abnormality. Lactase deficiency usually produces symptoms only in adulthood, although lactase levels in affected persons start to decline during childhood.[49] Lactase activity persists in most adults of western European heritage.[57] Even in this group, the activity of lactase is only approximately half the activity of sucrase and less than 20% of the activity of maltase.[58] Accordingly, in these persons, lactase activity is much more susceptible to a reduction in mucosal digestive function with acute or chronic GI illnesses.

In lactose malabsorbers, it may be unclear whether lactose malabsorption is from acquired primary lactase deficiency or is secondary to another small bowel disorder.[48] Therefore, in the individual lactose malabsorber, especially with an ethnic background associated with a low prevalence of acquired primary lactase deficiency, it may be necessary to exclude other malabsorptive small bowel disorders, such as celiac disease, as a cause of secondary lactase deficiency.

The main symptoms of lactose intolerance are bloating, abdominal cramps, increased flatus, and diarrhea. The development of bloating and abdominal cramps is associated with increased perception of luminal distention by gas.[59] Symptoms caused by distention of the colon or rectum by gas are not only related to the total volume of gas but also to the rate of gas accumulation. Reproducibility of symptoms is poor at lower distension volumes and becomes only good at higher distension volumes.[60]

No clear relation has been observed between the amount of lactose ingested and the severity of symptoms.[59,61] Ingestion of as little as 3 g of lactose to as much as 96 g of lactose may be required to induce symptoms in persons with lactose malabsorption.[61,62] GI symptoms, including diarrhea, have been shown to be more severe in adults with shorter small bowel transit time,[63] but no such relation between intestinal transit and symptoms has been observed in children.[64] In pregnant women[65] and in thyrotoxic patients with Graves disease,[66] changes in intestinal motility play a role in the clinical manifestation of lactose malabsorption.

In view of the poor correlation between lactose malabsorption and lactose intolerance, it is very important to monitor symptoms during a lactose hydrogen breath test, to confirm that symptoms during the test are truly representative of the patient's symptoms; that means that lactose malabsorption is associated with lactose intolerance.

Patients in whom a clear association between symptoms and lactose malabsorption can be established should be educated about a lactose-reduced diet. A lactose-free diet is rarely necessary. It is more important for the individual patient to learn his or her individual tolerance threshold, the amount of lactose that can be ingested without causing symptoms. If symptoms persist on a lactose-restricted diet, other substrates for colonic bacterial metabolism such as dietary fibers or fructose have to be restricted as well. Although patients sometimes question the use of drugs that contain lactose as an inactive ingredient, the amount of lactose contained in these drugs is usually so small that it does not cause symptoms.

Yogurt may be better tolerated by these patients,[67] and these products provide a good source of calcium. Consumption of whole milk or chocolate milk, rather than skim milk, and drinking milk with meals, may reduce symptoms of lactose intolerance, presumably as a result of prolongation of gastric emptying. Alternatively, supplementation of dairy products with lactase of microbiologic origin may be suggested.[68] Furthermore, persistence of some symptoms while the patient is on a lactose-free diet is not uncommon, because many carbohydrates other than lactose are incompletely absorbed by the normal small intestine[14] and because dietary fiber also may be metabolized by colonic bacteria. It also must be kept in mind that symptoms arising after ingestion of dairy products may instead be due to milk protein allergy or to intolerance of fat.

INCOMPLETE ABSORPTION AND INTOLERANCE OF FRUCTOSE (FRUCTOSE MALABSORPTION)

Fructose is found in modern diets either as a constituent of the disaccharide sucrose or as the monosaccharide, used as a sweetener in a variety of food items. Average daily intake varies from 11 to 54 g.[69] Fructose as a constituent of sucrose is absorbed by a well-characterized absorptive system integrating enzymatic hydrolysis of the disaccharide by sucrase and transfer of the resulting 2 monosaccharides through the apical membrane of the epithelial cell. The absorptive capacity for fructose that is not accompanied by glucose, however, is relatively small.[70] The normal absorption capacity of fructose depends on other nutrients as well, and is poorly understood. Healthy subjects have the capacity to absorb up to 25 g of fructose, whereas many have incomplete absorption and intolerance with intake of 50 g of fructose.[71]

Ingestion of food that contains fructose in excess of glucose may result in symptoms such as abdominal bloating or diarrhea[72,73] and also may provoke symptoms in patients with irritable bowel syndrome.[74] It has been suggested that as little as 3 g of fructose may precipitate symptoms in functional bowel disorders. Gender may influence fructose malabsorption.[75] It remains unclear whether there is adaptation of symptoms to regular consumption of fructose.

Incomplete fructose absorption usually is identified by a positive result on a breath hydrogen test after ingestion of 25 or 50 g of fructose. Because fructose content in fruit and in soft drinks usually is below 8 g/100 g of fruit or drink, the amounts of fructose used in the breath hydrogen test are unphysiologic, and no data are available on how many asymptomatic people would have a positive test result. However, fructose contents of 30– to 40 g/100 g can be present in chocolate, caramel, and pralines.[76]

In a group of patients with isolated fructose malabsorption, no defect of the gene encoding the luminal fructose transporter (GLUT5) could be detected.[77] It is therefore unlikely that patients who present with GI symptoms really have a defect of intestinal fructose absorption; it is more likely that they belong to a self-selected subset of people in whom ingestion of foods rich in fructose provokes symptoms related to other disorders, such as irritable bowel syndrome, and who present for evaluation of possible incomplete fructose absorption. Patients in whom symptoms develop after ingestion of fructose-rich food also may represent a subset of persons with unique, but not necessarily abnormal, colonic bacterial activity.[78]

A placebo-controlled study on patients with incomplete fructose absorption in the authors' unit, which is currently submitted for publication, has shown that ingestion of the enzyme xylose isomerase, which catalyzes the reversible isomerization of glucose and fructose decreases area under the breath hydrogen curve, pain, and nausea after ingestion of a watery fructose load. Future studies will have to evaluate whether this effect is also present during ingestion of carbohydrate mixtures or food containing fructose, and persists over a lengthy observation period. (Komericki P, Akkilic-Materna M, Strimitzer T, et al. Oral xylose-isomerase decreases breath hydrogen excretion and improves gastrointestinal symptoms in fructose malabsorption: a randomized, double-blind, placebo-controlled trial. Submitted for publication.)

In conclusion, testing for fructose malabsorption by the hydrogen breath test may be useful in identifying a subset of patients in whom dietary restriction of foods with excessive fructose content may be beneficial in the treatment of bloating and diarrhea, although low doses of fructose may be difficult to exclude from diet.[79] Symptoms in these persons probably are the result of ingestion of unphysiologic amounts of fructose[73] and not the consequence of a defect in fructose absorption.

DISACCHARIDASE DEFICIENCIES AND TRANSPORT DEFECTS FOR MONOSACCHARIDES

Sucrase-isomaltase deficiency is an inborn deficiency of this intestinal brush border enzyme. Affected infants usually become symptomatic after weaning with the introduction of starch and sucrose to the diet. Symptoms and signs include osmotic diarrhea, failure to thrive, excess flatus, and occasional vomiting. The diagnosis can be established by an oral sucrose absorption test. Treatment includes dietary avoidance of starch and sucrose.[80] Patients with this disease tend to experience spontaneous resolution of their symptoms with age.

Trehalase deficiency results in malabsorption of the disaccharide trehalose (present in mushrooms), resulting in diarrhea or vomiting after ingestion of mushrooms.[80]

Glucose–galactose malabsorption is an inborn defect of the brush border sodium–glucose cotransporter (SGLT1). These patients suffer from neonatal onset of severe diarrhea, leading to dehydration in the first days of life. Diarrhea stops only if glucose and galactose are eliminated from the diet. Older children and adults tolerate the offending carbohydrates better, but the transport defect is lifelong. The diagnosis can be established with an oral glucose tolerance test or by in vitro glucose absorption tests performed on intestinal biopsy specimens. Therapy consists of a fructose-based diet free of glucose and galactose. After the age of 3 months, the addition of foods containing low quantities of glucose or galactose (eg, vegetables, fruits, cheese) is considered to be safe.[81]

DIAGNOSIS OF CARBOHYDRATE MALABSORPTION

The hydrogen breath test is a noninvasive test that takes advantage of the fact that in most people, bacterial carbohydrate metabolism results in accumulation of hydrogen, which then is absorbed by the colonic mucosa and excreted in breath. Using different carbohydrates, such as lactose or fructose, the hydrogen breath test can be used to detect malabsorption of the respective carbohydrates. Unfortunately, a considerable proportion of the population, 18% of persons in a study in people of European descent,[82] are hydrogen nonexcretors. In these persons, hydrogen breath test results may be falsely negative, because hydrogen is metabolized by bacteria to methane. These limitations and pitfalls of breath hydrogen testing have to be taken into account when test results are interpreted.[83]

The hydrogen breath test is considered to be positive for lactose malabsorption if an increase in breath hydrogen concentration of greater than 20 parts per million over baseline occurs after ingestion of 20 to 50 g of lactose. An increase within the first 30 minutes after ingestion of lactose has to be disregarded, because it may be due to bacterial degradation of lactose in the oral cavity. Up to 4 hours may be required for the increase in breath hydrogen concentration to occur. Breath hydrogen measurements obtained before and at 30, 60, 90, 180, and 240 minutes after ingestion of 50 g of lactose provide the best diagnostic yield, with the least possible number of measurements.[82]

Variable doses have also been used for evaluating incomplete fructose absorption by hydrogen test in different laboratories. This may have contributed to the authors' observation in a recent study that could not confirm incomplete fructose absorption in 19 of 65 patients who had a positive fructose hydrogen breath test within the preceeding year. (Komericki P, Akkilic-Materna M, Strimitzer T, et al. Oral xylose-isomerase decreases breath hydrogen excretion and improves gastrointestinal symptoms in fructose malabsorption: a randomized, double-blind, placebo-controlled trial. Submitted for publication.)

The lactose hydrogen breath test is considered to be the gold standard for the clinical evaluation of lactose malabsorption by many researchers, but this test may miss the disorder in hydrogen nonexcretors; in a population with a prevalence of 18% of hydrogen nonexcretion, the sensitivity of breath hydrogen test cannot be better than 82%.[82] In hydrogen nonexcretors, a breath methane measurement or a lactose tolerance test, that is, measurement of blood glucose before and 30 minutes after ingestion of 50 g of lactose, can be used. An increase in glucose concentration of <20 mg/dL over baseline within 30 minutes of ingestion of 50 g of lactose is indicative of lactose malabsorption. The lactose tolerance test has a lower sensitivity to diagnose lactose malabsorption compared with the lactose hydrogen breath test, but combination of lactose hydrogen breath test with lactose tolerance test increased sensitivity of the combined tests to 94%.[82]

A gene test has been validated in a population of European descent for the detection of primary lactase deficiency (adult-type hypolactasia). In these populations a single-nucleotide polymorphism (SNP) -13910 T/C upstream of the LPH gene is involved in the regulation of intestinal lactase expression.[52] The CC genotype at the SNP-13910 T/C is associated with acquired primary lactase deficiency (adult-type hypolactasia), whereas TC and TT genotypes are linked with lactase persistence.[50] This polymorphism can be used as a diagnostic test for adult-type hypolactasia.[53]

Stool tests can be used in patients with diarrhea. Results of studies in normal subjects who ingested lactulose or sorbitol have suggested that a fecal pH lower than 5.5 can serve as a qualitative indicator of carbohydrate malabsorption.[84] However, studies in patients with diarrhea after ingestion of lactose reported by Steffer and colleagues reported elsewhere in this issue have shown that 80% of these patients do not have fecal pH lower than 5.5. Fecal short-chain fatty acids and carbohydrates can be determined by gas chromatography.[8–11] Fecal carbohydrates can be also measured by the anthrone method, which measures carbohydrates on a weight basis.[4–6] By contrast, the reducing sugar method gives results on a molar basis and therefore provides information about the osmotic activity of malabsorbed carbohydrates.[3,7] Total organic acids (short chain fatty acids and lactic acid) can be measured in stool by titration.[4,12]

SUMMARY

Several effects influence the clinical manifestation of diarrhea in carbohydrate malabsorption. First, carbohydrates result in a dose-dependent acceleration of colonic transit, primarily in the proximal but also in the distal colon. Second, stool weight in carbohydrate malabsorption is correlated to colonic transit, but it is primarily influenced by the unabsorbed osmotic load of carbohydrates and short chain fatty acids. Third, stool consistency is influenced both by stool composition (carbohydrates, organic acids, electrolytes) and transit in the distal colon. Fourth, at similar stool weight, colonic transit is significantly slower during carbohydrate malabsorption as compared with colonic volume load of other origins.

To assess osmotic activity and the role of carbohydrate malabsorption for the pathogenesis of diarrhea, the sum of carbohydrates plus organic acids plus obligated cations has to be calculated. In diarrhea with only slightly increased stool weight, organic acids and electrolytes are the main driving force of carbohydrate-induced osmotic diarrhea. Only in severe carbohydrate malabsorption, with stool weight in excess of 500 g/d, does fecal carbohydrate excretion become a driving force.

Short chain fatty acids inhibit colonic transit. Since these acids are metabolic products of bacterial metabolism of dietary fibers, this effect on transit deserves further evaluation for a possible clinical role in the pathogenesis and treatment of slow-transit constipation. Treatment failure of dietary fibers could be related to inhibitory effects of short chain fatty acids on transit in some susceptible patients.

Diarrhea associated with antibiotics may result from inhibition of colonic salvage of incompletely absorbed carbohydrates; this may result in osmotic diarrhea or in deficiency of short chain fatty acids, which are an energy source for colonic mucosal cells.

In view of the poor correlation between lactose malabsorption and lactose intolerance, it is very important to monitor symptoms during a lactose hydrogen breath test, to confirm that symptoms during the test are truly representative of the patient's symptoms. In patients with lactose intolerance, a clear association between symptoms and lactose malabsorption has to be established, and the patient has to establish his or her individual tolerance threshold. If symptoms persist on a lactose-restricted diet, other substrates for colonic bacterial metabolism, like dietary fibers or fructose, have to be restricted as well.

Ingestion of xylose isomerase with fructose-containing food may in the future become a treatment option for symptoms of incomplete fructose absorption.

REFERENCES

1. Miller TL, Wolin MJ. Fermentations by saccharolytic intestinal bacteria. Am J Clin Nutr 1979;32:164–72.
2. Ruppin H, Bar Meir S, Soergel KH, et al. Absorption of short chain fatty acids by the colon. Gastroenterology 1980;78:1500–7.
3. Hammer HF, Fine KD, Santa Ana CA, et al. Carbohydrate malabsorption: its measurement and its contribution to diarrhea. J Clin Invest 1990;86:1936–44.
4. Hammer HF, Santa Ana CA, Schiller LR, et al. Studies of osmotic diarrhea induced in normal subjects by ingestion of polyethyleneglycol and lactulose. J Clin Invest 1989;84:1056–62.
5. Ameen VZ, Powell GK. A simple spectrophotometric method for quantitative fecal carbohydrate measurement. Clin Chim Acta 1985;152:3–9.
6. Ameen VZ, Powell GK, Jones LA. Quantitation of fecal carbohydrate excretion in patients with short bowel syndrome. Gastroenterology 1987;92:493–500.
7. Nelson N. A photometric adaption of the Somogyi method for the determination of glucose. J Biol Chem 1944;153:375–80.
8. Benson JR, Woo DJ. Polymeric columns for liquid chromatography. J Chromatogr Sci 1984;22:386–99.
9. Delahunty T, Hollander D. Liquid–chromatographic method for estimating urinary sugars: applicability to studies of intestinal permeability. Clin Chem 1986;32:1542–4.
10. Ross LF, Chapital DC. Simultaneous determination of carbohydrates and products of carbohydrate metabolism in fermentation mixtures by HPLC. J Chromatogr Sci 1987;25:112–7.
11. Fritz E, Hammer HF, Lipp RW, et al. Effects of lactulose and polyethylene glycol on colonic transit. Aliment Pharmacol Ther 2005;21:259–68.
12. Collin DP, McCormick PG. Determination of short chain fatty acids in stool ultrafiltrate and urine. Clin Chem 1974;20:1173–80.
13. Nightingale JM, Lennard-Jones JE, Gertner DJ, et al. Colonic preservation reduces need for parenteral therapy, increases incidence of renal stones, but does not change high prevalence of gall stones in patients with short bowel. Gut 1992;33:1493–7.
14. Stephen AM, Phillips SF. Passage of carbohydrate into the colon. Direct measurements in humans. Gastroenterology 1983;85:589–95.
15. Cummings JH, Macfarlane GT. Role of intestinal bacteria in nutrient metabolism. JPEN J Parenter Enteral Nutr 1997;21:357–65.
16. Hammer HF. Colonic hydrogen absorption: quantification of its effect on hydrogen accumulation caused by bacterial fermentation of carbohydrates. Gut 1993;34:818–22.
17. Basilisco G, Phillips SF. Colonic salvage in health and disease. Eur J Gastroenterol Hepatol 1993;5:777–83.
18. Hammer HF, Sheikh MS. Colonic gas excretion in induced carbohydrate malabsorption—effect of simethicone. Eur J Gastroenterol Hepatol 1992;4:141–5.
19. Göranzon H, Forsum E. Metabolizable energy in humans in two diets containing different sources of dietary fiber. Calculations and analysis. J Nutr 1987;117:267–73.

20. Florent C, Flourie B, Leblond A, et al. Influence of chronic lactulose ingestion on the colonic metabolism of lactulose in man (an in vivo study). J Clin Invest 1985; 75:608–13.

21. Yang MG, Manoharan K, Mickelsen O. Nutritional contribution of volatile fatty acids from the cecum of rats. J Nutr 1970;100:545–50.

22. Jeppesen PB, Mortensen PB. Significance of a preserved colon for parenteral energy requirements in patients receiving home parenteral nutrition. Scand J Gastroenterol 1998;33:1175–9.

23. Moore JG, Jessop LD, Osborne DN. A gas chromatographic and mass spectrometric analysis of the odor of human feces. Gastroenterology 1987;93:1321–9.

24. El-Yamani J, Mizon C, Capon C, et al. Decreased faecal exoglycosidase activities identify a subset of patients with active Crohn's disease. Clin Sci (Lond) 1992;83: 409–15.

25. Rao SS, Read NW, Holdsworth CD. Is the diarrhoea in ulcerative colitis related to impaired colonic salvage of carbohydrate? Gut 1987;28:1090–4.

26. Högenauer C, Hammer HF, Krejs GJ, et al. Mechanisms and management of antibiotic-associated diarrhea. Clin Infect Dis 1998;27:702–10.

27. Kurpad AV, Shetty PS. Effects of antimicrobial therapy on faecal bulking. Gut 1986;27:55–8.

28. Roediger WE. Role of anaerobic bacteria in the metabolic welfare of the colonic mucosa in man. Gut 1980;21:793–8.

29. Roediger WE. The colonic epithelium in ulcerative colitis: an energy-deficiency disease? Lancet 1980;2:712–5.

30. Harig JM, Soergel KH, Komorowski RA, et al. Treatment of diversion colitis with short-chain fatty acid irrigation. N Engl J Med 1989;320:23–8.

31. Edwards CA, Duerden BI, Read NW. Effect of clindamycin on the ability of a continuous culture of colonic bacteria to ferment carbohydrate. Gut 1986;27:411–7.

32. Rao SS, Edwards CA, Austen CJ, et al. Impaired colonic fermentation of carbohydrate after ampicillin. Gastroenterology 1988;94:928–32.

33. Finegold SM. Interaction of antimicrobial therapy and intestinal flora. Am J Clin Nutr 1970;23:1466–71.

34. Bjorneklett A, Midtvedt T. Influence of three antimicrobial agents—penicillin, metronidazole and doxycyclin—on the intestinal microflora of healthy humans. Scand J Gastroenterol 1981;16:473–80.

35. Clausen MR, Bonnen H, Tvede M, et al. Colonic fermentation to short-chain fatty acids is decreased in antibiotic-associated diarrhea. Gastroenterology 1991;101: 1497–504.

36. Hove H, Tvede M, Brobech-Mortensen P. Antibiotic-associated diarrhoea, *Clostridium difficile*, and short-chain fatty acids. Scand J Gastroenterol 1996;31: 688–93.

37. Hammer J, Pruckmayer M, Bergmann H, et al. The distal colon provides reserve storage capacity during colonic fluid overload. Gut 1997;41:658–63.

38. Flourié B, Briet F, Florent C, et al. Can diarrhea induced by lactulose be reduced by prolonged ingestion of lactulose? Am J Clin Nutr 1993;58:369–75.

39. Hammer J, Phillips SF. Fluid loading of the human colon: effects on segmental transit and stool composition. Gastroenterology 1993;105:988–98.

40. Debongnie JC, Phillips SF. Capacity of the human colon to absorb fluid. Gastroenterology 1978;74:698–703.

41. Jouët P, Sabate JM, Flourie B, et al. Effects of therapeutic doses of lactulose vs. polyethylene glycol on isotopic colonic transit. Aliment Pharmacol Ther 2008;27: 988–93.

42. Squires PE, Rumsey RD, Edwards CA, et al. Effect of short chain fatty acids on contractile activity and fluid flow in rat colon in vitro. Am J Physiol 1992;262: G813–7.
43. Ashraf W, Park F, Lof J, et al. Effects of psyllium therapy on stool characteristics, colon transit and anorectal function in chronic idiopathic constipation. Aliment Pharmacol Ther 1995;9:639–47.
44. Odstrcil EA, Martinez JG, Santa Ana CA, et al. The contribution of malabsorption to the reduction in net energy absorption after long-limb Roux-en-Y gastric bypass. Am J Clin Nutr 2010;92:704–13.
45. Layer P, Go VL, DiMagno EP. Fate of pancreatic enzymes during small intestinal aboral transit in humans. Am J Physiol 1986;251:G475–80.
46. Antonowicz I, Lebenthal E. Developmental patterns of small intestinal enterokinase and disaccharidase activities in the human fetus. Gastroenterology 1977; 72:1299–303.
47. Savilahti E, Launiala K, Kuitunen P. Congenital lactase deficiency: a clinical study on 16 patients. Arch Dis Child 1983;58:246–52.
48. Barrett JS, Irving PM, Shepherd SJ, et al. Comparison of the prevalence of fructose and lactose malabsorption across chronic intestinal disorders. Aliment Pharmacol Ther 2009;30:165–74.
49. Welsh JD, Poley JR, Bhatia M, et al. Intestinal disaccharidase activities in relation to age, race, and mucosal damage. Gastroenterology 1978;75:847–55.
50. Johnson JD. The regional and ethnic distribution of lactose malabsorption: adaptive and genetic hypotheses. In: Paige DM, Bayless TM, editors. Lactose digestion: clinical and nutritional implications. Baltimore (MD): Johns Hopkins University Press; 1981. p. 11–22.
51. Sahi T. Genetics and epidemiology of adult-type hypolactasia. Scand J Gastroenterol Suppl 1994;202:7–20.
52. Troelsen JT, Olsen J, Moller J, et al. An upstream polymorphism associated with lactase persistence has increased enhancer activity. Gastroenterology 2003;125: 1686–94.
53. Escher JC, de Koning ND, van Engen CG, et al. Molecular basis of lactase levels in adult humans. J Clin Invest 1992;89:480–3.
54. Enattah NS, Sahi T, Savilahti E, et al. Identification of a variant associated with adult-type hypolactasia. Nat Genet 2002;30:233–7.
55. Högenauer C, Hammer HF, Mellitzer K, et al. Evaluation of a new DNA test compared with the lactose hydrogen breath test for the diagnosis of lactase non-persistence. Eur J Gastroenterol Hepatol 2005;17:371–6.
56. Ingram CJ, Elamin MF, Mulcare CA, et al. A novel polymorphism associated with lactose tolerance in Africa: multiple causes for lactase persistence? Hum Genet 2007;120:779–88.
57. Enattah NS, Jensen TG, Nielsen M, et al. Independent introduction of two lactase-persistence alleles into human populations reflects different history of adaptation to milk culture. Am J Hum Genet 2008;82:57–72.
58. Sterchi EE, Mills PR, Fransen JA, et al. Biogenesis of intestinal lactase-phlorizin hydrolase in adults with lactose intolerance. J Clin Invest 1990;86:1329–37.
59. Hammer HF, Petritsch W, Pristautz H, et al. Evaluation of the pathogenesis of flatulence and abdominal cramps in patients with lactose malabsorption. Wien Klin Wochenschr 1996;108:175–9.
60. Hammer HF, Phillips SF, Camilleri M, et al. Rectal tone, distensibility and mechanoperception: intraindividual reproducibility and responses to different distension protocols. Am J Physiol 1998;274(3 Pt 1):G584–90.

61. Gudmand-Hoyer E, Simony K. Individual sensitivity to lactose in lactose malabsorption. Am J Dig Dis 1977;22:177–81.
62. Bedine MS, Bayless TM. Intolerance of small amounts of lactose by individuals with low lactase levels. Gastroenterology 1973;65:735–43.
63. Ladas SD, Papanikos J, Arapakis G. Lactose malabsorption in Greek adults: correlation of small bowel transit time with the severity of lactose intolerance. Gut 1982;23:968–73.
64. Roggero P, Offredi ML, Mosca F, et al. Lactose absorption and malabsorption in healthy italian children: do the quantity of malabsorbed sugar and the small bowel transit time play a role in symptom production? J Pediatr Gastroenterol Nutr 1985;4:82–6.
65. Szilagyi A, Salomon R, Martin M, et al. Lactose handling by women with lactose malabsorption is improved during pregnancy. Clin Invest Med 1996;19:416–26.
66. Szilagyi A, Lerman S, Barr RG, et al. Reversible lactose malabsorption and intolerance in Graves' disease. Clin Invest Med 1991;14:188–97.
67. Kolars JC, Levitt MD, Aouji M, et al. Yogurt: an autodigesting source of lactose. N Engl J Med 1984;310:1–3.
68. Moskovitz M, Curtis C, Gavaler J. Does oral enzyme replacement therapy reverse intestinal lactose malabsorption? Am J Gastroenterol 1987;82:632–5.
69. Gibson PR, Newnham E, Barrett JS, et al. Review article: fructose malabsorption and the bigger picture. Aliment Pharmacol Ther 2007;25:349–63.
70. Jones HF, Butler RN, Brooks DA. Intestinal fructose transport and malabsorption in humans. Am J Physiol Gastrointest Liver Physiol 2011;300:G202–6.
71. Rao SS, Attaluri A, Anderson L, et al. Ability of the normal human small intestine to absorb fructose: evaluation by breath testing. Clin Gastroenterol Hepatol 2007;5: 959–63.
72. Hoekstra JH, van-Kempen AA, Kneepkens CM. Apple juice malabsorption: fructose or sorbitol? J Pediatr Gastroenterol Nutr 1993;16:39–42.
73. Beyer PL, Caviar EM, McCallum RW. Fructose intake at current levels in the United States may cause gastrointestinal distress in normal adults. J Am Diet Assoc 2005;105:1559–66.
74. Evans PR, Piesse C, Bak YT, et al. Fructose-sorbitol malabsorption and symptom provocation in irritable bowel syndrome: relationship to enteric hypersensitivity and dysmotility. Scand J Gastroenterol 1998;33:1158–63.
75. Szilagyi A, Malolepszy P, Yesovitch S, et al. Fructose malabsorption may be gender dependent and fails to show compensation by colonic adaptation. Dig Dis Sci 2007;52:2999–3004.
76. Mishkin D, Sablauskas L, Yalovsky M, et al. Fructose and sorbitol malabsorption in ambulatory patients with functional dyspepsia: comparison with lactose maldigestion/malabsorption. Dig Dis Sci 1997;42:2591–8.
77. Wasserman D, Hoekstra JH, Tolia V, et al. Molecular analysis of the fructose transporter gene (GLUT5) in isolated fructose malabsorption. J Clin Invest 1996;98: 23198–402.
78. Born P, Zech J, Lehn H, et al. Colonic bacterial activity determines the symptoms in people with fructose-malabsorption. Hepatogastroenterology 1995;42:778–85.
79. Kyaw MH, Mayberry JF. Fructose malabsorption: true condition or a variance from normality. J Clin Gastroenterol 2011;45:16–21.
80. Semenza G, Auricchio S, Mantei N, et al. Small-intestinal disaccharidases. In: Scriver CR, Beaudet AL, Sly WS, et al, editors. The metabolic and molecular bases of inherited diseases. 8th edition. New York: McGraw-Hill; 2001. p. 1623–50.

81. Wright EM, Martin MG, Turk E, et al. Familial glucose-galactose malabsorption and hereditary renal glycosuria. In: Scriver CR, Beaudet AL, Sly WS, et al, editors. The metabolic and molecular bases of inherited diseases. 8th edition. New York: McGraw-Hill; 2001. p. 4891–907.

82. Hammer HF, Petritsch W, Pristautz H, et al. Assessment of the influence of hydrogen nonexcretion on the usefulness of the hydrogen breath test and lactose tolerance test. Wien Klin Wochenschr 1996;108:137–41.

83. Simren M, Stotzer PO. Use and abuse of hydrogen breath tests. Gut 2006;55: 297–303.

84. Eherer AJ, Fordtran JS. Fecal osmotic gap and pH in experimental diarrhea of various causes. Gastroenterology 1992;103:545–51.

Functional Diarrhea

Jan Tack, MD, PhD

KEYWORDS

- Chronic diarrhea • Functional diarrhea • Irritable bowel syndrome
- Rapid intestinal transit

KEY POINTS

- Chronic diarrhea, specifically functional diarrhea, is a clinical problem of considerable magnitude.
- The epidemiology of this condition needs further studies, because the overlap with diarrhea-predominant irritable bowel syndrome (D-IBS) is usually not taken into account in currently available literature.
- The role of stress and of specific nutrient intolerances is incompletely elucidated.
- In clinical practice, a stepwise diagnostic approach can be used to eliminate underlying organic disease in a cost-effective fashion. A similar approach can be used to identify and eliminate potential precipitating or worsening food constituents.
- Although there are many available pharmacologic treatment options that can be used in these patients, comparative studies establishing a hierarchy of cost benefit and a sequence of use of such agents are lacking.

INTRODUCTION AND DEFINITION

Chronic diarrhea is a frequent presenting symptom, seen by both general practitioners and gastroenterologists. The differential diagnosis is broad, and diagnostic evaluation may be complex.[1–3]

In spite of the large number of causes of chronic diarrhea, and in spite of extensive investigations, no cause for the symptoms is found in a large group of patients, who are referred to as having functional diarrhea.[3]

According to the Rome III Diagnostic Criteria for Functional Gastrointestinal Disorders (Rome III criteria), functional diarrhea is defined as the presence of loose (mushy) or watery stools in at least 75% of stools, in the absence of pain. The presence of pain distinguishes functional diarrhea from D-IBS. In addition, the symptoms have to be chronic, with an onset of at least 6 months before diagnosis and active symptoms during the prior 3 months.[3]

Competing interests: None declared.
Department of Clinical and Experimental Medicine, Translational Research Center for Gastrointestinal Disorders (TARGID), University of Leuven, Herestraat 49, Leuven B-3000, Belgium
E-mail address: jan.tack@med.kuleuven.ac.be

Gastroenterol Clin N Am 41 (2012) 629–637
http://dx.doi.org/10.1016/j.gtc.2012.06.007
0889-8553/12/$ – see front matter © 2012 Published by Elsevier Inc.

gastro.theclinics.com

The Rome III criteria used stool consistency rather than frequency or the presence of urgency for the definition of functional diarrhea. This definition is based on the association of stool consistency with transit times and on the possibility for urgency to occur even in the presence of solid stools.[3,4] Alternatively, frequency and the presence of urgency are important components of self-reported diarrhea in patients and in the general population.[5]

EPIDEMIOLOGY

The prevalence of functional diarrhea in the population is poorly studied. Most available surveys on the epidemiology of chronic diarrhea have not systematically distinguished D-IBS from other types of chronic diarrhea, and in a condition with such a broad differential diagnosis, symptom-based criteria are insufficient to exclude several organic causes. Nevertheless, a telephone survey in the United States found that 26.9% of 1017 respondents reported symptoms of diarrhea or loose stools in the prior month, with similar prevalences in both genders.[6] The definition used in this survey, however, was less stringent than the Rome III consensus definitions.

A recent survey in Olmsted County, Minnesota, studied the prevalence of chronic diarrhea and excluded irritable bowel syndrome (IBS) based on Rome III criteria.[7] In a questionnaire mailed to 892 eligible subjects, 73% responded, with 28% reporting chronic diarrhea. In 60% of these, the diarrhea was painless, and this was associated with self-reported food intolerance and with stress and was less prevalent in women and in those with a higher education. Chronic diarrhea was not associated with age, marital status, body mass index, smoking history, acetaminophen, aspirin, nonsteroidal anti-inflammatory drugs, coffee use, alcohol use, pets, or water supply. The definition used (≥3 bowel movements a day, loose or watery stools, or fecal urgency on at least 25% of the occasions), however, was still less stringent than the Rome III definition for functional diarrhea.[3] In addition, the study could not correct for identifiable causes, such as lactose intolerance and celiac disease, although their impact is likely low.

DIAGNOSTIC APPROACH

History taking should evaluate the ingestion of poorly absorbed carbohydrates (fructose, sorbitol, and so forth), which may cause diarrhea, or a link between symptoms and ingestion of dairy products, suggestive of lactose intolerance. The Bristol stool form scale can be used as a visual aid to confirm a patient's usual stool consistency. Medication use needs to be assessed, because several drugs (magnesium-containing antacids; lipase inhibitors, such as orlistat; prokinetics, such as erythromycin and metoclopramide; colchicine; misoprostil; and broad-spectrum antibiotics) may cause diarrhea as an adverse effect.

The presence of abdominal pain (suggestive of IBS or other causes), weight loss (suggestive of malabsorption), steatorrhea-like stools or nocturnal diarrhea, recent intake of antibiotics or a history of abdominal surgery all argue in favor of other specific diagnoses and should be evaluated. Similarly, a family history of inflammatory bowel disease, celiac disease, or colorectal cancer should increase suspicion of organic disorders. Physical examination should evaluate abdominal or rectal masses, signs of anemia, and signs of malnutrition (edema, skin or nail abnormalities, and so forth).[1-3] Digital rectal examination should assess anal sphincter tone.

Chronic diarrhea generally requires additional technical examinations, including blood work with assessment of C-reactive protein, signs of malabsorption, thyroid function, and celiac disease screening. Colonoscopy is recommended in those above 50 years old and those with a recent onset of symptoms, but the threshold for ordering ileocolonoscopy (exclusion of polyps or inflammatory bowel disease) with biopsies (exclusion of microscopic colitis) and upper endoscopy with duodenal biopsies (exclusion of giardiasis and villous atrophy) is low in patients with chronic diarrhea. In refractory cases, analysis of 3-day stool collection volume and composition, tests for bile acid malabsorption, and small bowel radiograph can be considered. Additional evaluations include tests for small intestinal bacterial overgrowth and screening for secretive (factitious) laxative use. Several diagnostic algorithms have been published, which allow identifying organic or specific causes of chronic diarrhea through a cost-effective sequence of investigations.[8,9]

PATHOPHYSIOLOGIC MECHANISMS IN FUNCTIONAL DIARRHEA

Although many studies have addressed pathophysiologic mechanisms in D-IBS, functional diarrhea is poorly studied. The stool consistency, which is a key feature in the Rome III definition of functional diarrhea, suggests that rapid bowel transit is present in patients with chronic diarrhea.[3,5] In keeping with an underlying motility disorder, a colonic manometry study found increased propagating colonic contractions and decreased nonpropagating contractions in functional diarrhea patients.[10]

Epidemiologic research found an association between chronic diarrhea and self-reported stress in the general population. A study in healthy volunteers confirmed that acute dichotomous listening stress enhances small bowel transit whereas gastric emptying times were not affected.[11] Chronic diarrhea, with or without abdominal pain, may be precipitated by an acute gastroenteritis, and in these patients falls within the spectrum of postinfectious bowel disorders.[12]

TREATMENT APPROACH

Clear explanation of the symptoms and diagnosis and reassurance about the benign nature of chronic functional diarrhoea are important. It is worthwhile to discuss potential triggering factors, such as specific foods, stress, and anxiety. Dietary restrictions of food components, such as fructose, sorbitol, caffeine, or other precipitating foods, are generally proposed as a first approach.[2,3,9] A trial of lactose elimination can be advocated in those who consume milk products on a regular basis.[13] In addition, restrictions of alcohol, which may precipitate diarrhea in susceptible subjects, and foods rich in fiber are recommended.[2,3,9] A diet-and-stool diary may help identify aggravating factors.[14]

Pharmacotherapy can be considered as a first-line treatment in those who have symptoms with major impact on their quality of life or can be added in those who fail to respond sufficiently to reassurance and dietary measures. Antidiarrheal agents may be classified as intestinal transit inhibitors (opioids, tricyclic antidepressants, and 5-HT$_3$ antagonists), intraluminal agents (cholestyramine, medicinal fiber, clays, activated charcoal, and bismuth), proabsorptive agents (clonidine), and antisecretory drugs (octreotide).

INTESTINAL TRANSIT INHIBITORS
Opioid Agonists

Opioid receptor ligands are the most frequently used agents in the (symptomatic) treatment of diarrhea. Morphine is well known to slow gastrointestinal transit and codeine, a μ-opioid receptor agonist, is less potent but also has antidiarrheal properties. Because of their central effects and risk of habituation, these opioids are usually avoided in the treatment of chronic diarrhea. Diphenoxylate and loperamide, especially, are preferentially used because they lack central nervous system effects.[15,16]

The drug most commonly used in clinical practice is loperamide, a peripherally acting μ-receptor agonist without addictive properties. Loperamide inhibits peristalsis and slows intestinal and colonic transit times, thereby allowing more complete absorption of electrolytes and water. In addition, loperamide increases anal sphincter pressure and reduces the sensitivity of the rectum to distention, which is beneficial in cases of associated urge incontinence.[17,18] Starting doses of loperamide are 2 mg to 4 mg, with titration to patient symptoms and stool pattern. A high interindividual dose variation exists, and in some patients with large volumes of liquid stool, doses may be increased up to 24 mg in divided doses over 24 hours. Loperamide can also be taken prophylactically before meals or when leaving the house.

Diphenoxylate is another μ-opioid agonist with peripheral actions similar to loperamide but which does cross the blood-brain barrier. To prevent overdosage, atropine is added to diphenoxylate capsules in some countries. In a crossover study with placebo in patients with chronic diarrhea, diphenoxylate with atropine significantly reduced stool frequency and daily stool weight.[19] Adverse effects related to diphenoxylate or to atropine have been reported.[20]

One trial comparing the efficacy of loperamide, codeine, and diphenoxylate plus atropine in patients with chronic diarrhea showed that loperamide or codeine were more efficacious and better tolerated than diphenoxylate.[21] Another study compared loperamide to the α_2-agonist, lidamidine, and to placebo in chronic diarrhea and found superior symptomatic responses to loperamide compared with lidamidine and placebo.[22] A placebo-controlled trial in fecal incontinence showed that loperamide improved urgency and urgency incontinence. This was associated with increased anal sphincter pressure and an improved capacity for rectal retention of fluids.[17]

5-HT₃ Receptor Antagonists

5-HT₃ receptor antagonists increase colonic transit times.[23,24] Clinical studies with the 5-HT₃ receptor antagonist, alosetron, showed improved stool pattern and relief of pain/discomfort in women with D-IBS at a dose of 1 mg twice a day.[25] The drug also improved symptoms of urgency and urgency incontinence in D-IBS.[26] Data regarding its efficacy in functional diarrhea not related to IBS are lacking, but based on the mode of action and based on clinical experience, the drug seems efficacious in this condition. Shortly after its introduction to the US market, however, alosetron was withdrawn because of side effects of colonic ischemia.[27] The drug was subsequently reintroduced in a restricted access program in the United States and follow-up reports have shown a good safety profile in this limited-use setting.[28] In Japan, the 5-HT3 receptor antagonist, ramosetron, has been approved for the treatment of D-IBS in men.[29,30]

Tricyclic Antidepressants

Tricyclic antidepressants have some anticholinergic and, therefore, antidiarrheal actions. In an uncontrolled study in patients with fecal incontinence, amitryptiline prolonged colonic transit time, improved stool consistency, suppressed rectal motor events, and improved fecal incontinence.[31] Desipramine was investigated in a large, multicenter, placebo-controlled study of IBS but showed only beneficial effects in a per protocol analysis, whereas the intention-to-treat failed to show benefit due to poor tolerance with a high number of discontinuations.[32] Because the study did not report details on stool pattern and urgency, it is unclear how well diarrhea symptoms responded.

Racecadotril

Racecadotril is an enkephalinase inhibitor, developed for the treatment of diarrhea. Clinical efficacy has mainly been established in acute infectious diarrhea. Studies comparing racecadotril to loperamide in adults with acute infectious diarrhea or in elderly patients residing in nursing homes with diarrhea reported rapid and complete resolution of diarrhea, with fewer symptoms of abdominal pain or constipation.[33,34] It is unclear whether the drug affects intestinal transit; a study with acetorphan, another enkephalinase inhibitor, showed no effect on transit.[35] Studies of enkephalinase inhibitors in functional diarrhea are lacking.

INTRALUMINAL AGENTS
Bile-Acid Binding Agents

Up to 50% of patients with chronic idiopathic diarrhea have bile acid malabsorption.[36-43] Studies report that this is the group of patients that responds best to cholestyramine treatment. Cholestyramine and related binding resins improve urgency and stool consistency and reduce stool frequency and stool weight.[39,44,45] The dose used is 4 g, up to 3 times daily, with the early morning dose considered the most important. Palatability and solubility of cholestyramine are problematic, but dissolving the drug in a glass of orange juice, which is refrigerated overnight, may mitigate these tolerance issues.

Bismuth

Bismuth subsalicylate has been shown effective in acute travelers' diarrhea; its effectiveness in chronic diarrhea has mainly been addressed in microscopic colitis,[46,47] and potential usefulness in other types of chronic diarrhea is unproved. Bismuth's effectiveness is thought to depend on some antisecretory action as well as antimicrobial properties. In theory, absorbion of bismuth may harbor potential risk of encephalopathy. For these reasons, chronic bismuth treatment cannot be recommended.

Bulking and Hydroscopic Agents

Bulking agents, such as psyllium, or hydroscopic agents, such as gum agar, are usually used in the treatment of constipation. By increasing stool bulk and by absorbing water and decreasing stool fluidity, however, they may aid in the treatment of mild diarrhea, especially fecal incontinence.[48,49] Although these agents may alter stool consistency, they do not reduce stool weight and are not suitable for patients with larger-volume diarrhea. The efficacy of fiber and gum agar in fecal incontinence was assessed in 2 studies, where improvement was associated with more formed stools.[48,49] One open crossover study compared loperamide with isphagula husk in chronic diarrhea and reported similar effects on stool frequency but less urgency and better stool consistency with ispaghula husk.[50] No controlled double-blind studies are available.

Other Treatments

AST-120 is a complex spherical carbon adsorbent that showed some signs of efficacy on abdominal pain and on stool consistency in a controlled pilot trial in D-IBS.[51] So far, no studies in functional diarrhea have been reported.

Probiotics are a vast new area of therapeutic investigation in gastrointestinal disorders and a rapidly expanding area of research. One study investigated the effects of lyophilized, heat-killed *Lactobacillus acidophilus* LB versus living lactobacilli in the treatment of chronic diarrhea.[52] Symptoms, including stool frequency, improved significantly more in the group receiving lyophilized, heat-killed *Lactobacillus acidophilus* LB, suggesting a potential role in the treatment of chronic diarrhea.

PROABSORPTIVE DRUGS: CLONIDINE

In diabetic diarrhea, efficacy of clonidine, a proabsorptive agent, in doses up to 300 μg, 3 times a day, has been reported.[53] The beneficial effects of clonidine probably also include motility components, because the drug was shown to slow intestinal transit and to inhibit colonic tone in health.[54,55] The efficacy of clonidine in nondiabetic chronic diarrhea has not been addressed. Taking into account the unfavorable side-effect profile, mainly due to hypotension and nausea, clonidine should be considered in patients who fail to respond to opiate agonist treatment. The dose should be gradually titrated up, starting from 75 μg twice a day, up to 150 μg 3 times a day. Lidamidine, a related α_2-agonist, was studied in chronic diarrhea but was reportedly inferior to loperamide.[22]

ANTISECRETORY DRUGS: OCTREOTIDE

The use of the somatostatin analog octreotide has been investigated in several types of chronic diarrhea, including carcinoid diarrhea, dumping syndrome, short bowel syndrome, chemotherapy-induced diarrhea, and AIDS-associated diarrhea.[56] Octreotide enhances intestinal absorption and inhibits gastric, pancreatic, and intestinal secretion. Favorable responses have been reported for diabetic diarrhea as well.[57]

Based on these properties, octreotide has been applied in the treatment of chronic idiopathic (functional) diarrhea, at doses ranging between 50 μg and 500 μg, 3 times a day.[58] Taking into account the cost and the mode of administration (subcutaneous injections 3 times a day), somatostatin analogs should be considered third-line agents, to be tried when more conventional treatments have failed.[58] Furthermore, chronic use may be complicated by gallstone formation and related complications.[59] Successful use of the slow-release formulation octreotide long-acting repeatable, administered intramuscularly on a monthly basis, has been reported for neuroendocrine tumor-related and chemotherapy-related diarrhea.[60,61]

SUMMARY

Chronic diarrhea, specifically functional diarrhea, is a clinical problem of considerable magnitude. The epidemiology of this condition needs further studies, because the overlap with D-IBS is usually not taken into account in currently available literature. The underlying pathophysiology may involve rapid intestinal transit, but only few quality mechanistic studies are available. The role of stress, and of specific nutrient intolerances, is incompletely elucidated. In clinical practice, a stepwise diagnostic approach can be used to eliminate underlying organic disease in a cost-effective fashion. A similar approach can be used to identify and eliminate potential precipitating or worsening food constituents. Although there are many available pharmacologic treatment options that can be used in these patients, comparative studies establishing a hierarchy of cost benefit and a sequence of use of such agents are lacking.

REFERENCES

1. Fine KD, Schiller LR. AGA technical review on the evaluation and management of chronic diarrhea. Gastroenterology 1999;116:1464–86.
2. Schiller LR. Chronic diarrhea. Gastroenterology 2004;127:287–93.
3. Longstreth GF, Thompson WG, Chey WD, et al. Functional bowel disorders. Gastroenterology 2006;130(5):1480–91.
4. Sandler RS, Drossman DA. Bowel habits in young adults not seeking health care. Dig Dis Sci 1987;32:841–5.

5. Lewis SJ, Heaton KW. Stool form scale as a useful guide to intestinal transit time. Scand J Gastroenterol 1997;32(9):920–4.
6. Sandler RS, Stewart WF, Liberman JN, et al. Abdominal pain, bloating, and diarrhea in the United States: prevalence and impact. Dig Dis Sci 2000;45(6):1166–71.
7. Chang JY, Locke GR 3rd, Schleck CD, et al. Risk factors for chronic diarrhoea in the community in the absence of irritable bowel syndrome. Neurogastroenterol Motil 2009;21(10):1060-e87.
8. Camilleri M. Chronic diarrhea: a review on pathophysiology and management for the clinical gastroenterologist. Clin Gastroenterol Hepatol 2004;2(3):198–206.
9. Spiller RC, Thompson WG. Bowel disorders. Am J Gastroenterol 2010;105(4): 775–85.
10. Bazzocchi G, Ellis J, Villanueva-Meyer J, et al. Effect of eating on colonic motility and transit in patients with functional diarrhea. Gastroenterology 1991;101: 1298–306.
11. Cann PA, Read NW, Cammack J, et al. Psychological stress and the passage of a standard meal through the stomach and small intestine in man. Gut 1983;24:236–40.
12. Spiller RC. Inflammation as a basis for functional GI disorders. Best Pract Res Clin Gastroenterol 2004;18(4):641–61.
13. Lomer MC, Parkes GC, Sanderson JD. Review article: lactose intolerance in clinical practice–myths and realities. Aliment Pharmacol Ther 2008;27(2):93–103.
14. Parker TJ, Naylor SJ, Riordan AM, et al. Management of patients with food intolerance in irritable bowel syndrome: the development and use of an exclusion diet. J Hum Nutr Diet 1995;8:159–66.
15. Lavo B, Stenstam M, Nielsen AL. Loperamide in treatment of irritable bowel syndrome—a double-blind placebo controlled study. Scand J Gastroenterol Suppl 1987;22:77–80.
16. Corazziari E. Role of opioid ligands in the irritable bowel syndrome. Can J Gastroenterol 1999;13(Suppl A):71A–5A.
17. Read M, Read NW, Barber DC, et al. Effects of loperamide on anal sphincter function in patients complaining of chronic diarrhoea with faecal incontinence and urgency. Dig Dis Sci 1982;27:807–14.
18. Sun WM, Read NW, Verlinden M. Effects of loperamide oxide on gastrointestinal transit time and anorectal function in patients with chronic diarrhoea and faecal incontinence. Scand J Gastroenterol 1997;32:34–8.
19. Gattuso JM, Kamm MA. Adverse effects of drugs used in the management of constipation and diarrhoea. Drug Saf 1994;10:47–65.
20. Harford WV, Krejs GJ, Santa Ana CA, et al. Acute effect of diphenoxylate with atropine (Lomotil) in patients with chronic diarrhoea and faecal incontinence. Gastroenterology 1980;78:440–3.
21. Palmer KR, Corbett CL, Holdsworth CD. Double-blind cross-over study comparing loperamide, codeine and diphenoxylate in the treatment of chronic diarrhoea. Gastroenterology 1980;79:1272–5.
22. Allison MC, Sercombe J, Pounder RE. A double-blind crossover comparison of lidamidine, loperamide and placebo for the control of chronic diarrhoea. Aliment Pharmacol Ther 1988;2:347–51.
23. Talley NJ, Phillips SF, Haddad A, et al. Effect of selective 5HT3 antagonist (GR38032F) on small intestinal transit and release of gastrointestinal peptides. Dig Dis Sci 1989;34:1511–5.
24. Thumshirn M, Coulie B, Camilleri M, et al. Effects of alosetron on gastrointestinal transit time and rectal sensation in patients with irritable bowel syndrome. Aliment Pharmacol Ther 2000;14(7):869–78.

25. Camilleri M, Northcutt AR, Kong SA, et al. Efficacy and safety of alosetron in women with irritable bowel syndrome: a randomised, placebo-controlled trial. Lancet 2000;355:1035–40.

26. Lembo AJ, Olden KW, Ameen VZ, et al. Effect of alosetron on bowel urgency and global symptoms in women with severe, diarrhea-predominant irritable bowel syndrome: analysis of two controlled trials. Clin Gastroenterol Hepatol 2004;2:675–82.

27. Thompson CA. Alosetron withdrawn from market. Am J Health Syst Pharm 2001; 58:13.

28. Chang L, Tong K, Ameen V. Ischemic colitis and complications of constipation associated with the use of alosetron under a risk management plan: clinical characteristics, outcomes, and incidences. Am J Gastroenterol 2010;105(4): 866–75.

29. Matsueda K, Harasawa S, Hongo M, et al. A phase II trial of the novel serotonin type 3 receptor antagonist ramosetron in Japanese male and female patients with diarrhea-predominant irritable bowel syndrome. Digestion 2008;77(3–4):225–35.

30. Lee KJ, Kim NY, Kwon JK, et al. Efficacy of ramosetron in the treatment of male patients with irritable bowel syndrome with diarrhea: a multicenter, randomized clinical trial, compared with mebeverine. Neurogastroenterol Motil 2011;23(12):1098–104.

31. Santoro GA, Eitan BZ, Pryde A, et al. Open study of low dose amitriptyline in the treatment of patients with idiopathic fecal incontinence. Dis Colon Rectum 2000; 43:1676–82.

32. Drossman DA, Toner BB, Whitehead WE, et al. Cognitive-behavioral therapy versus education and desipramine versus placebo for moderate to severe functional bowel disorders. Gastroenterology 2003;125:19–31.

33. Prado D, Global Adult Racecadotril Study Group. A multinational comparison of racecadotril and loperamide in the treatment of acute watery diarrhoea in adults. Scand J Gastroenterol 2002;37:656–61.

34. Gallelli L, Colosimo M, Tolotta GA, et al. Prospective randomized double-blind trial of racecadotril compared with loperamide in elderly people with gastroenteritis living in nursing homes. Eur J Clin Pharmacol 2010;66(2):137–44.

35. Bergmann JF, Chaussade S, Couturier D, et al. Effects of acetorphan, an antidiarrhoeal enkephalinase inhibitor, on oro-caecal and colonic transit times in healthy volunteers. Aliment Pharmacol Ther 1992;6(3):305–13.

36. Sciarretta G, Vicini G, Fagioli G, et al. Use of 23-selena-25-homocholyltaurine to detect bile acid malabsorption in patients with ileal dysfunction or diarrhea. Gastroenterology 1986;91:1–9.

37. Sciarretta G, Fagioli G, Furno A, et al. 75Se HCAT test in the detection of bile acid malabsorption in functional diarrhoea and its correlation with small bowel transit. Gut 1987;28:970–5.

38. Suhr O, Danielsson A, Nyhlin H, et al. Bile acid malabsorption demonstrated by SeHCAT in chronic diarrhoea, with special reference to the impact of cholecystectomy. Scand J Gastroenterol 1988;23:1187–94.

39. Williams AJ, Merrick MV, Eastwood MA. Idiopathic bile acid malabsorption—a review of clinical presentation, diagnosis, and response to treatment. Gut 1991;32:1004–6.

40. Eusufzai S. Bile acid malabsorption in patients with chronic diarrhoea. Scand J Gastroenterol 1993;28:865–8.

41. Rudberg U, Nylander B. Radiological bile acid absorption test 75SeHCAT in patients with diarrhoea of unknown cause. Acta Radiol 1996;37:672–5.

42. Niaz SK, Sandrasegaran K, Renny FH, et al. Postinfective diarrhoea and bile acid malabsorption. J R Coll Physicians Lond 1997;31:53–6.

43. Wildt S, Norby Rasmussen S, Lysgard Madsen J, et al. Bile acid malabsorption in patients with chronic diarrhoea: clinical value of SeHCAT test. Scand J Gastroenterol 2003;38:826–30.

44. Duncombe VM, Bolin TD, Davis AE. Double-blind trial of cholestyramine in post-vagotomy diarrhoea. Gut 1977;18:531–5.

45. Sinha L, Liston R, Testa HJ, et al. Idiopathic bile acid malabsorption: qualitative and quantitative clinical features and response to cholestyramine. Aliment Pharmacol Ther 1998;12:839–44.

46. Fine KD, Lee EL. Efficacy of open-label bismuth subsalicylate for the treatment of microscopic colitis. Gastroenterology 1998;114:29–36.

47. Fine KD, Ogunji F, Lee E. Randomized, double-blind, placebo controlled trial of bismuth subsalicylate for microscopic colitis [abstract]. Gastroenterology 1999; 116:A880.

48. Chassagne P, Jego A, Gloc P, et al. Does treatment of constipation improve faecal incontinence in institutionalized elderly patients? Age Ageing 2000;29: 159–64.

49. Bliss DZ, Jung HJ, Savik K, et al. Supplementation with dietary fiber improves fecal incontinence. Nurs Res 2001;50:203–13.

50. Qvitzau S, Matzen P, Madsen P. Treatment of chronic diarrhoea: loperamide versus ispaghula husk and calcium. Scand J Gastroenterol 1988;23:1237–40.

51. Tack JF, Miner PB Jr, Fischer L, et al. Randomised clinical trial: the safety and efficacy of AST-120 in non-constipating irritable bowel syndrome - a double-blind, placebo-controlled study. Aliment Pharmacol Ther 2011;34(8):868–77.

52. Xiao SD, Zhang DZ, Lu H, et al. Multicenter, randomized, controlled trial of heat-killed Lactobacillus acidophilus LB in patients with chronic diarrhea. Adv Ther 2003;20:253–60.

53. Fedorak RN, Field M, Chang EB. Treatment of diabetic diarrhea with clonidine. Ann Intern Med 1985;102:197–9.

54. Rubinoff MJ, Piccione PR, Holt PR. Clonidine prolongs human small intestine transit time: use of the lactulose-breath hydrogen test. Am J Gastroenterol 1989;84:372–4.

55. Viramontes BE, Malcolm A, Camilleri M, et al. Effects of an alpha(2)-adrenergic agonist on gastrointestinal transit, colonic motility, and sensation in humans. Am J Physiol Gastrointest Liver Physiol 2001;281:G1468–76.

56. Farthing MJ. Octreotide in the treatment of refractory diarrhoea and intestinal fistulae. Gut 1994;35(Suppl 3):S5–10.

57. Valdovinos MA, Camilleri M, Zimmerman BR. Chronic diarrhea in diabetes mellitus: mechanisms and an approach to diagnosis and treatment. Mayo Clin Proc 1993;68:691–702.

58. Fried M. Octreotide in the treatment of refractory diarrhea. Digestion 1999; 60(Suppl 2):42–6.

59. Redfern JS, Fortuner WJ 2nd. Octreotide-associated biliary tract dysfunction and gallstone formation: pathophysiology and management. Am J Gastroenterol 1995;90:1042–52.

60. Rosenoff S. Resolution of refractory chemotherapy-induced diarrhea (CID) with octreotide long-acting formulation in cancer patients: 11 case studies. Support Care Cancer 2004;12:561–70.

61. Ricci S, Antonuzzo A, Galli L, et al. Octreotide acetate long-acting release in patients with metastatic neuroendocrine tumors pretreated with lanreotide. Ann Oncol 2000;11:1127–30.

Celiac Disease

Kate E. Evans, MRCP[a],*, David S. Sanders[b,c]

KEYWORDS

- Celiac disease • Diarrhea • Gluten • Diet • Small bowel

KEY POINTS

- Celiac disease affects 1% of the population but the diagnosis is often missed or delayed.
- Serology is inadequate for diagnosis; a small-bowel biopsy should demonstrate villous atrophy.
- Up to one-third of patients have persisting symptoms, usually because of inadvertent gluten ingestion.
- Conditions associated with chronic diarrhea in celiac disease include microscopic colitis, pancreatic insufficiency, small bowel bacterial overgrowth, and lactose intolerance.
- Refractory celiac disease is rare. Selected cases may respond to immunosuppression.

CONTEMPORARY CELIAC DISEASE

Celiac disease is defined as a state of heightened immunologic responsiveness to ingested gluten in genetically susceptible individuals.[1] Epidemiologic studies screening cohorts of healthy adult volunteers in the United States, United Kingdom, and other European countries consistently report a prevalence of 0.5% to 1.0%.[2–4] There is some evidence that the prevalence is increasing.[5–7] Despite being a common, global phenomenon, diagnosis is often delayed.[8,9]

Definitions

The first diagnostic criteria for celiac disease by the European Society of Pediatric Gastroenterology and Nutrition in 1969 required a structurally abnormal mucosa while taking gluten, a clear improvement in villous structure while on gluten-free diet (GFD), and relapse of the mucosal changes on gluten challenge.[10] This 3-step approach

The authors have nothing to disclose.
[a] Department of Gastroenterology and Liver Unit, Royal Hallamshire Hospital, Room P39, Sheffield, South Yorkshire, S10 2JF, UK; [b] Department of Gastroenterology and Liver Unit, Royal Hallamshire Hospital, Sheffield, South Yorkshire, S10 2JF, UK; [c] University of Sheffield, Room P39, Sheffield, South Yorkshire, S10 2JF, UK
* Corresponding author.
E-mail address: kateemmaevans@hotmail.com

reflects the thinking of the day that celiac disease was a permanent condition that started in childhood. The subsequent 40 years have seen an evolution in endoscopy, the development of highly accurate serologic tests, and large epidemiologic studies that have contributed to our current understanding of celiac disease. It is now recognized that most patients may have more subtle presenting symptoms, adult presentations are more frequent than pediatric, and there is a "pre-celiac" state.[4,11]

Recognition of the celiac iceberg has improved understanding and detection of celiac disease (**Fig. 1**).[9] The visible iceberg above the waterline depicts patients with typical gastrointestinal symptoms, such as diarrhea and weight loss. The subsequent stratum just below the waterline represents patients considered to have atypical presentations. They may have vague, nonspecific gastrointestinal symptoms, such as bloating, or conditions associated with celiac disease, such as iron deficiency anemia, osteoporosis, and persistently abnormal liver function tests.[12–14] Patients are often identified in screening groups, which would include those with type 1 diabetes, autoimmune thyroid disease, or a first-degree relative with celiac disease.

The deeper layers of the iceberg represent the "pre-celiac" state. Latent celiac disease describes a patient with a normal small bowel mucosa while on a gluten-containing diet who later develops celiac disease. It has been shown that before the development of villous atrophy, some patients may have symptoms, such as abdominal pain, weight loss, and diarrhea, or complications, such as osteoporosis.[15–20] Furthermore, these may resolve with GFD.[17–19,21] Latent celiac disease also describes the converse situation: a patient with biopsy-proven celiac disease who later has a normal small-bowel biopsy despite a normal, gluten-containing diet. One recent study found that 13 of 61 adults with biopsy-proven celiac disease in childhood now following a normal diet had normal mucosa at repeat biopsy.[22] Two of the 13 with latent disease relapsed at subsequent follow-up. In this carefully selected group, up to 18% may have true latency and immune tolerance to gluten.

Recently, the National Institutes of Health consensus group used the term latent celiac disease to describe individuals with positive serology and normal biopsy and

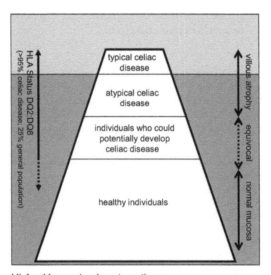

HLA = Human Leukocyte antigen.

Fig. 1. The "celiac iceberg." HLA, HLA antigen.

this has been adopted by some researchers.[23] The term "potential celiac disease" can also be used to describe positive serology with normal biopsy. This may be found in first-degree relatives of patients with celiac disease,[3] as well as those with autoimmune diseases, such as hypothyroidism. The term gluten sensitivity may be used interchangeably with potential celiac disease and is defined as a condition of some morphologic, immunologic, or functional disorder that responds to gluten exclusion.[17] This includes gluten-sensitive diarrhea and immunologic response to gluten in family members of celiac patients.[24]

DIAGNOSIS

As demonstrated by the celiac iceberg, the presence of relevant symptoms or serologic testing alone is not sufficient to confirm the diagnosis. A simple diagnostic algorithm is shown in **Fig. 2**.

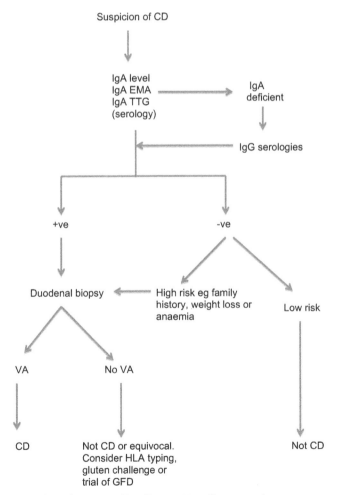

Fig. 2. Diagnostic algorithm. CD, celiac disease; VA, villous atrophy.

Serology

Endomysial antibody (EMA) and tissue transglutaminase (TTG) have a combined sensitivity and specificity of more than 90% when used in combination in selected, high celiac prevalence populations.[25] However, when the prevalence of celiac disease falls to 1%, as found in screening populations, the positive predictive value of these tests falls to approximately 80% or less.[26] The sensitivity of the serologic tests also falls well below 90% when histologic grades less than Marsh 3 (villous atrophy) are considered.[27–29] This is a clinical problem that is difficult to evaluate, as most studies have excluded patients without villous atrophy.[30] Pooled data for diagnostic accuracy of serologic testing is therefore precluded by the heterogeneous nature of the studies. Instead, ranges for sensitivity and specificity are given in **Table 1**.[31] It is also important to note that there is no linear relationship between adherence to GFD, mucosal recovery, and serology. It is possible to have normalization of serology with persisting villous atrophy.[32] Likewise, a clinical response to GFD is not predictive of mucosal recovery.[33] Indeed, although most patients report a subjective improvement on GFD, complete mucosal recovery may occur in only 8% of patients.[34] Serology alone is inadequate for diagnosis.[31] False-positive TTG occurs in conditions such as inflammatory bowel disease, autoimmune disease, and chronic liver disease.[35] Conversely antibody-negative disease accounts for about 9% (4%–22%) of cases.[25,36–38] Causes of antibody-negative celiac disease include selective immunoglobulin A (IgA) deficiency, immunosuppressive therapy, and self-imposed gluten-free diet.[39] Of course the possibility that the villous atrophy is not caused by celiac disease must also be considered.

A new class of assays detecting the presence of antibodies to deamidated synthetic peptides of gliadin has shown high diagnostic performance equivalent to conventional tests.[40–42] A recent meta-analysis does not suggest any diagnostic advantage is conferred by the use of these newer assays.[43] Likewise, point-of-care testing (fingerprick testing) has shown early promise but currently lacks the sensitivity and specificity required to replace conventional serology.[44,45]

HLA

A negative test for HLA DQ2 and DQ8 has a high negative predictive value and is useful to exclude celiac disease. This may have a role in those with borderline histology or serology, unwilling to give up a self-imposed GFD, or with a family history.[46–48] HLA status may also be used to risk stratify first-degree relatives. Based on a gene dose effect, clinicians in the future may be able to quantify the risk of developing celiac disease to be low or high depending on the presence or absence of homozygosity.[49,50]

Biopsy

The patchy nature of the histologic change in celiac disease is well documented.[51–53] For this reason, it is recommended to take multiple small-bowel biopsies to minimize sampling error.[47] Since the advent of fiberoptic endoscopy, biopsies are usually taken

Table 1
Sensitivity and specificity of celiac serologies

Test	Sensitivity Range, %	Specificity Range, %
IgA EMA	68–100	89–100
IgA TTG	38–100	25–100
IgA a-DGP	79–98	80–95

Abbreviations: a-DGP, anti-deamidated gliadin peptides; EMA, endomysial antibody; IgA, immunoglobulin A; TTG, tissue transglutaminase.

from the second part of the duodenum. This has been shown to be equivalent to jejunal biopsy for the detection of villous atrophy.[54] A recent advance in this field is the demonstration that optimal strategies for diagnosing celiac disease can only achieve 100% sensitivity by always including a duodenal bulb biopsy.[25,53,55,56] Historically, bulb biopsy was avoided because of a belief that Brunner glands interfered with interpretation of atrophy.[57] However, this belief is not evidence based. In one prospective study, 9% (n = 126) of adults with newly diagnosed celiac disease had villous atrophy in the bulb only.[56] No control patient had villous atrophy in the bulb alone. Furthermore, causes of villous atrophy other than celiac disease are rare. Non-celiac villous atrophy should be considered in "nonresponsive celiac disease" and causes include peptic inflammation, *Giardia*, *Helicobacter* infection, and Crohn disease.[25,57,58] Histologic grades that fall short of villous atrophy, ie, Marsh grade 1 and 2, are a gray area. There is some evidence that suggests this situation should be managed as celiac disease with villous atrophy. One group randomized 23 patients with positive EMA, compatible HLA status, and Marsh grade 1 or 2 changes to receive either normal diet or GFD.[59] Those on GFD had improvement symptomatically, serologically, and histologically. Those on normal diet showed persistence or worsening of all parameters. This finding is supported by others.[60] However, caution should be exercised because these lesser changes are not uncommon and are not always attributable to celiac disease.[61] Other causes include drugs, immune dysregulation, and infection.[61,62]

DIARRHEA IN CELIAC DISEASE

Although it is increasingly recognized that celiac disease can present without gastrointestinal symptoms, diarrhea remains a common presenting complaint.[8,13] One large survey included 2681 adults with biopsy-proven celiac disease.[63] In this study, the most common, self-reported presenting symptoms included abdominal pain (83%), diarrhea (76%), and weight loss (69%). Screening populations could be expected to have fewer symptoms than health care–seeking individuals, although the astute physician may identify symptoms and signs.[44] In one primary care screening study, 976 patients were investigated and celiac disease was diagnosed in 22 patients. Of these, 6 of 22 had unexplained chronic diarrhea.[64]

Nonresponsive Celiac Disease

Nonresponsive celiac disease (NRCD) has historically been described as failure to respond to a GFD. This can be primary NRCD (ie, an individual who never responded to a GFD) or a subsequent recurrence of symptoms after 1 year (secondary NRCD).[65] Contemporary clinical studies suggest that NRCD occurs in about 17% to 30%.[14,66,67] Most cases of NRCD are related to either inadvertent ingestion of tiny, but clinically significant amounts of gluten or nonadherence.[66,68,69]

In the patient with NRCD, it is important to challenge the initial diagnosis of celiac disease. In one reported series of 55 patients referred for NRCD, the original diagnosis of celiac disease was disproved in 6.[69] All previous diagnostic investigations including the serology and duodenal biopsies should all be reviewed. Biopsies should be reviewed by a specialist gastrointestinal pathologist. Supportive evidence should be sought in the form of compatible HLA status (DQ2 or DQ8), a positive family history of celiac disease, or functional hyposplenism.

Gluten Exposure

Adherence to a GFD is estimated to be in the order of 42% to 91% based on self-reporting.[70–73] The most common reason for NRCD is continued gluten exposure. In one study of patients with celiac disease and persisting symptoms, 25 of 49 were identified as having gluten contamination responsible for their ongoing clinical and histologic signs.[69] Inadvertent ingestion usually occurred in the form of commercially packaged cereals derived from corn or rice that had contained malted barley. Adherence is best assessed by a skilled dietician.

Associated Conditions

There are other causes of chronic diarrhea in patients with celiac disease who are adherent to a GFD.[66,69,74] Diagnoses associated with celiac disease include microscopic colitis, pancreatic insufficiency, irritable bowel syndrome (IBS), small bowel bacterial overgrowth, thyroid dysfunction, and secondary intolerances (owing to mucosal surface damage, for example, lactose or fructose intolerance).[66] Microscopic colitis is more common in patients with celiac disease than in controls without celiac disease. One recent large population-based study found an incidence of microscopic colitis in celiac disease 50 times that in the general population.[75] The association most often occurred in middle-aged women. Diagnosis requires pan-colonic biopsies.[76,77] Pancreatic abnormalities are associated with celiac disease.[67,78] One study of patients with celiac disease and chronic diarrhea found that almost one-third (20/666) had low fecal pancreatic elastase levels. Furthermore, pancreatic supplementation conferred some benefit with a reduction in stool frequency.[67]

IBS can mimic the symptoms of celiac disease and it is recommended that patients presenting with IBS are tested for celiac disease.[79–81] Small bowel bacterial overgrowth is recognized as a cause of persisting symptoms in celiac disease. In one study of 15 patients with persisting symptoms, 10 showed small intestinal bacterial overgrowth by lactulose breath test. When these patients were treated with antibiotics (rifaximin) after 1 month, they were symptom free[60]; however, antibiotic therapy does not always improve symptoms and breath tests may not reliably identify those who will respond.[82] Adult autoimmune enteropathy is recognized as a rare cause of villous atrophy. Patients have severe enteropathy unresponsive to any exclusion diet and are positive for enterocyte antibodies.[83,84]

Refractory Celiac Disease

The normal small intestinal intraepithelial lymphocyte (IEL) population is composed of approximately 80% to 85% CD8+ T-cell receptor (TCR)$\alpha\beta$ cells and 15% CD8+TCR$\gamma\delta$ cells. In uncomplicated celiac disease, IELs express CD3+ and CD8+ (T suppressor/cytotoxic phenotype) and there is an increase in $\gamma\delta$ T cells. Celiac disease may be regarded as refractory (RCD) when symptoms persist (primary) or recur (secondary) despite the adherence to a strict GFD and when other causes have been excluded.[65] RCD is subdivided into types I and II with a phenotypically normal or aberrant intraepithelial T-cell population respectively.[85] This is determined by using polymerase chain reaction analysis for the TCR gene rearrangement. Quantification in percentage terms is used as a means of differentiating RCD I from RCD II. Patients with RCD I have less than 10% of aberrant (clonal) T cells on duodenal biopsy.[85] This differentiation helps in prognostication. RCD I is more likely to respond to immunosuppression, whereas RCD II seems largely resistant to treatment, and transition to enteropathy-associated T-cell lymphoma (EATL) is common. Although ulcerative jejunitis and EATL remain rare complications of celiac disease overall, they are relatively common in a subset of patients with RCD II.[86,87] In one study of 93 patients with RCD, 43 had RCD I and none had celiac-related mortality at 5 years. In the group with RCD II (n = 50), the overall 5-year survival was 58%, falling to 8% in the 26 (52%) who developed EATL.[86] A recent study has demonstrated that the aberrant immunophenotype and monoclonality may be transiently detected in patients with celiac disease who are not adherent, however; thus, it is important not just to take a snapshot but to have repeat testing.[87]

Typically, RCD presents with severe malnutrition, malabsorption, hypoalbuminemia, and weight loss.[88] Weight loss can be predictive of refractory CD.[68] HLADQ2 homozygous patients appear more likely to develop secondary EATL or de novo EATL.[86] Therapeutic options are limited but there is some evidence that azathioprine and prednisolone (or budesonide) may confer benefit in RCD I.[89] For type II refractory disease and/or EATL, many other treatments, including cyclosporine, interleukin-10, elemental diet, alemtuzumab, cladribine, CHOP (a combination of doxorubicin, cyclophosphamide, vincristine, and prednisolone), and autologous stem cell transplantation have been described in case series.[87] It is beyond the scope of this review to give further detail.

SUMMARY

In conclusion, up to one-third of patients with celiac disease will have persistent symptoms. Most cases will be related to adherence aspects of their GFD. In patients with persisting symptoms, after reaffirming the diagnosis of celiac disease, it is important to differentiate between those with adherence issues or associated conditions, such as bacterial overgrowth, and those with true refractory celiac disease. By doing this, specific associated diseases can be diagnosed and treated. If these other causes have been excluded and the patient has true refractory disease, RCD I and II should be clearly delineated. This allows the clinician an opportunity to provide the patient with important prognostic information and determine who may respond to immunosuppression (RCD I). We recommend early nutritional supplementation and even enteral or parenteral nutrition if appropriate. The prognosis for RCD II remains poor but there a number of novel therapies currently being evaluated.

REFERENCES

1. American Gastroenterological Association medical position statement: Celiac Sprue. Gastroenterology 2001;120(6):1522–5.
2. West J, Logan RF, Hill PG, et al. Seroprevalence, correlates, and characteristics of undetected coeliac disease in England. Gut 2003;52(7):960–5.
3. Fasano A, Berti I, Gerrarduzzi T, et al. Prevalence of celiac disease in at-risk and not-at-risk groups in the United States: a large multicenter study. Arch Intern Med 2003;163(3):286–92.
4. Green PH, Jabri B. Coeliac disease. Lancet 2003;362(9381):383–91.
5. Catassi C, Kryszak D, Bhatti B, et al. Natural history of celiac disease autoimmunity in a USA cohort followed since 1974. Ann Med 2010;42(7):530–8.
6. Lohi S, Mustalahti K, Kaukinen K, et al. Increasing prevalence of coeliac disease over time. Aliment Pharmacol Ther 2007;26(9):1217–25.
7. Rubio-Tapia A, Kyle RA, Kaplan EL, et al. Increased prevalence and mortality in undiagnosed celiac disease. Gastroenterology 2009;137(1):88–93.
8. Green PH. The many faces of celiac disease: clinical presentation of celiac disease in the adult population. Gastroenterology 2005;128(4 Suppl 1): S74–8.
9. Fasano A, Catassi C. Current approaches to diagnosis and treatment of celiac disease: an evolving spectrum. Gastroenterology 2001;120(3):636–51.
10. Meeuwisse G. Diagnostic criteria in coeliac disease. Acta Paediatr Scand 1970; 59:461–3.

11. Ferguson A, Arranz E, O'Mahony S. Clinical and pathological spectrum of coeliac disease—active, silent, latent, potential. Gut 1993;34(2):150–1.
12. Sanders DS, Carter MJ, Hurlstone DP, et al. Association of adult coeliac disease with irritable bowel syndrome: a case-control study in patients fulfilling ROME II criteria referred to secondary care. Lancet 2001;358(9292):1504–8.
13. Sanders DS, Hurlstone DP, Stokes RO, et al. Changing face of adult coeliac disease: experience of a single university hospital in South Yorkshire. Postgrad Med J 2002;78(915):31–3.
14. Green PHR, Stavropoulos SN, Panagi SG, et al. Characteristics of adult celiac disease in the USA: results of a national survey. Am J Gastroenterol 2001; 96(1):126–31.
15. Ludvigsson JF, Michaelsson K, Ekbom A, et al. Coeliac disease and the risk of fractures—a general population-based cohort study. Aliment Pharmacol Ther 2007;25(3):273–85.
16. Ludvigsson JF, Brandt L, Montgomery SM. Symptoms and signs in individuals with serology positive for celiac disease but normal mucosa. BMC Gastroenterol 2009;9:57.
17. Mustalahti K, Collin P, Sievänen H, et al. Osteopenia in patients with clinically silent coeliac disease warrants screening. Lancet 1999;354(9180):744–5.
18. Dickey W, Hughes DF, McMillan SA. Patients with serum IgA endomysial antibodies and intact duodenal villi: clinical characteristics and management options. Scand J Gastroenterol 2005;40(10):1240–3.
19. Kaukinen K, Mäki M, Partanen J, et al. Celiac disease without villous atrophy: revision of criteria called for. Dig Dis Sci 2001;46(4):879–87.
20. Kaukinen K, Peräaho M, Collin P, et al. Small-bowel mucosal transglutaminase 2-specific IgA deposits in coeliac disease without villous atrophy: a prospective and randomized clinical study. Scand J Gastroenterol 2005;40(5):564–72.
21. Scott BB, Losowsky MS. Coeliac disease with mild mucosal abnormalities: a report of four patients. Postgrad Med J 1977;53(617):134–8.
22. Matysiak-Budnik T, Malamut G, de Serre NP, et al. Long-term follow-up of 61 coeliac patients diagnosed in childhood: evolution toward latency is possible on a normal diet. Gut 2007;56(10):1379–86.
23. James SP. This month at the NIH: Final statement of NIH Consensus Conference on celiac disease. Gastroenterology 2005;128(1):6.
24. Troncone R, Franzese A, Mazzarella G, et al. Gluten sensitivity in a subset of children with insulin dependent diabetes mellitus. Am J Gastroenterol 2003;98(3): 590–5.
25. Hopper AD, Cross SS, Hurlstone DP, et al. Pre-endoscopy serological testing for coeliac disease: evaluation of a clinical decision tool. BMJ 2007;334(7596):729.
26. Hill ID. What are the sensitivity and specificity of serologic tests for celiac disease? Do sensitivity and specificity vary in different populations? Gastroenterology 2005;128(4 Suppl 1):S25–32.
27. Tursi A, Giorgetti G, Brandimarte G, et al. Prevalence and clinical presentation of subclinical/silent celiac disease in adults: an analysis on a 12-year observation. Hepatogastroenterology 2001;48(38):462–4.
28. Tursi A, Brandimarte G, Giorgetti GM. Prevalence of antitissue transglutaminase antibodies in different degrees of intestinal damage in celiac disease. J Clin Gastroenterol 2003;36(3):219–21.
29. Rostami K, Kerckhaert J, Tiemessen R, et al. Sensitivity of antiendomysium and antigliadin antibodies in untreated celiac disease: disappointing in clinical practice. Am J Gastroenterol 1999;94(4):888–94.

30. Lewis NR, Scott BB. Systematic review: the use of serology to exclude or diagnose coeliac disease (a comparison of the endomysial and tissue transglutaminase antibody tests). Aliment Pharmacol Ther 2006;24(1):47–54.
31. Evans KE, Sanders DS. What is the use of biopsy and antibodies in coeliac disease diagnosis? J Intern Med 2011;269(6):572–81.
32. Hopper AD, Hadjivassiliou M, Hurlstone DP, et al. What is the role of serologic testing in celiac disease? A prospective, biopsy-confirmed study with economic analysis. Clin Gastroenterol Hepatol 2008;6(3):314–20.
33. Rubio-Tapia A, Rahim MW, See JA, et al. Mucosal recovery and mortality in adults with celiac disease after treatment with a gluten-free diet. Am J Gastroenterol 2010;105(6):1412–20.
34. Lanzini A, Lanzarotto F, Villanacci V, et al. Complete recovery of intestinal mucosa occurs very rarely in adult coeliac patients despite adherence to gluten-free diet. Aliment Pharmacol Ther 2009;29(12):1299–308.
35. Vecchi M, Folli C, Donato MF, et al. High rate of positive anti-tissue transglutaminase antibodies in chronic liver disease. Role of liver decompensation and of the antigen source. Scand J Gastroenterol 2003;38(1):50–4.
36. Tursi A, Brandimarte G, Giorgetti G, et al. Low prevalence of antigliadin and anti-endomysium antibodies in subclinical/silent celiac disease. Am J Gastroenterol 2001;96(5):1507–10.
37. Dickey W, Hughes DF, McMillan SA. Reliance on serum endomysial antibody testing underestimates the true prevalence of coeliac disease by one fifth. Scand J Gastroenterol 2000;35(2):181–3.
38. Salmi TT, Collin P, Korponay-Szabó IR, et al. Endomysial antibody-negative coeliac disease: clinical characteristics and intestinal autoantibody deposits. Gut 2006;55(12):1746–53.
39. Cataldo F, Marino V, Ventura A, et al. Prevalence and clinical features of selective immunoglobulin A deficiency in coeliac disease: an Italian multicentre study. Italian Society of Paediatric Gastroenterology and Hepatology (SIGEP) and "Club del Tenue" Working Groups on Coeliac Disease. Gut 1998;42(3):362–5.
40. Volta U, Granito A, Parisi C, et al. Deamidated gliadin peptide antibodies as a routine test for celiac disease: a prospective analysis. J Clin Gastroenterol 2010;44(3):186–90.
41. Sugai E, Nachman F, Váquez H, et al. Dynamics of celiac disease-specific serology after initiation of a gluten-free diet and use in the assessment of compliance with treatment. Dig Liver Dis 2010;42(5):352–8.
42. Niveloni S, Sugai E, Cabanne A, et al. Antibodies against synthetic deamidated gliadin peptides as predictors of celiac disease: prospective assessment in an adult population with a high pretest probability of disease. Clin Chem 2007;53(12):2186–92.
43. Lewis NR, Scott BB. Meta-analysis: deamidated gliadin peptide antibody and tissue transglutaminase antibody compared as screening tests for coeliac disease. Aliment Pharmacol Ther 2010;31(1):73–81.
44. Korponay-Szabo IR, Szabados K, Pusztai J, et al. Population screening for coeliac disease in primary care by district nurses using a rapid antibody test: diagnostic accuracy and feasibility study. BMJ 2007;335(7632):1244–7.
45. Ferre-López S, Ribes-Koninckx C, Genzor C, et al. Immunochromatographic sticks for tissue transglutaminase and antigliadin antibody screening in celiac disease. Clin Gastroenterol Hepatol 2004;2(6):480–4.
46. Kaukinen K, Partanen J, Mäki M, et al. HLA-DQ typing in the diagnosis of celiac disease. Am J Gastroenterol 2002;97(3):695–9.

47. Rostom A, Murray JA, Kagnoff MF. American Gastroenterological Association (AGA) Institute technical review on the diagnosis and management of celiac disease. Gastroenterology 2006;131(6):1981–2002.

48. Bonamico M, Ferri M, Mariani P, et al. Serologic and genetic markers of celiac disease: a sequential study in the screening of first degree relatives. J Pediatr Gastroenterol Nutr 2006;42(2):150–4.

49. Cassinotti A, Birindelli S, Clerici M, et al. HLA and autoimmune digestive disease: a clinically oriented review for gastroenterologists. Am J Gastroenterol 2009; 104(1):195–217 [quiz: 194, 218].

50. Bourgey M, Calcagno G, Tinto N, et al. HLA related genetic risk for coeliac disease. Gut 2007;56(8):1054–9.

51. Green PH. Celiac disease: how many biopsies for diagnosis? Gastrointest Endosc 2008;67(7):1088–90.

52. Ravelli A, Villanacci V, Monfredini C, et al. How patchy is patchy villous atrophy?: distribution pattern of histological lesions in the duodenum of children with celiac disease. Am J Gastroenterol 2010;105(9):2103–10.

53. Weir DC, Glickman JN, Roiff T, et al. Variability of histopathological changes in childhood celiac disease. Am J Gastroenterol 2010;105(1):207–12.

54. Mee AS, Burke M, Vallon AG, et al. Small bowel biopsy for malabsorption: comparison of the diagnostic adequacy of endoscopic forceps and capsule biopsy specimens. Br Med J (Clin Res Ed) 1985;291(6498):769–72.

55. Corazza GR, Villanacci V, Zambelli C, et al. Comparison of the interobserver reproducibility with different histologic criteria used in celiac disease. Clin Gastroenterol Hepatol 2007;5(7):838–43.

56. Evans KE, Aziz I, Cross SS, et al. A prospective study of duodenal bulb biopsy in newly diagnosed and established adult celiac disease. Am J Gastroenterol 2011; 106(10):1837–42.

57. Shidrawi RG, Przemioslo R, Davies DR, et al. Pitfalls in diagnosing coeliac disease. J Clin Pathol 1994;47(8):693–4.

58. Evans KE, Sanders DS. Joint BAPEN and British Society of Gastroenterology Symposium on 'Coeliac disease: basics and controversies'. Coeliac disease: optimising the management of patients with persisting symptoms? Proc Nutr Soc 2009;68(3):242–8.

59. Kurppa K, Collin P, Viljamaa M, et al. Diagnosing mild enteropathy celiac disease: a randomized, controlled clinical study. Gastroenterology 2009;136(3): 816–23.

60. Tursi A, Brandimarte G. The symptomatic and histologic response to a gluten-free diet in patients with borderline enteropathy. J Clin Gastroenterol 2003;36(1): 13–7.

61. Biagi F, Bianchi PI, Campanella J, et al. The prevalence and the causes of minimal intestinal lesions in patients complaining of symptoms suggestive of enteropathy: a follow-up study. J Clin Pathol 2008;61(10):1116–8.

62. Aziz I, Evans KE, Hopper AD, et al. A prospective study into the aetiology of lymphocytic duodenosis. Aliment Pharmacol Ther 2010;32(11–12):1392–7.

63. Cranney A, Zarkadas M, Graham ID, et al. The Canadian Celiac Health Survey. Dig Dis Sci 2007;52(4):1087–95.

64. Catassi C, Kryszak D, Louis-Jacques O, et al. Detection of celiac disease in primary care: a multicenter case-finding study in North America. Am J Gastroenterol 2007;102(7):1454–60.

65. Ryan BM, Kelleher D. Refractory celiac disease. Gastroenterology 2000;119(1): 243–51.

66. Fine KD, Meyer RL, Lee EL. The prevalence and causes of chronic diarrhea in patients with celiac sprue treated with a gluten-free diet. Gastroenterology 1997;112(6):1830–8.
67. Leeds JS, Hopper AD, Hurlstone DP, et al. Is exocrine pancreatic insufficiency in adult coeliac disease a cause of persisting symptoms? Aliment Pharmacol Ther 2007;25(3):265–71.
68. Leffler DA, Dennis M, Hyett B, et al. Etiologies and predictors of diagnosis in nonresponsive celiac disease. Clin Gastroenterol Hepatol 2007;5(4):445–50.
69. Abdulkarim AS, Burgart LJ, See J, et al. Etiology of nonresponsive celiac disease: results of a systematic approach. Am J Gastroenterol 2002;97(8):2016–21.
70. Hall NJ, Rubin G, Charnock A. Systematic review: adherence to a gluten-free diet in adult patients with coeliac disease. Aliment Pharmacol Ther 2009;30(4): 315–30.
71. Häuser W, Gold J, Stein J, et al. Health-related quality of life in adult coeliac disease in Germany: results of a national survey. Eur J Gastroenterol Hepatol 2006;18(7):747–54.
72. Leffler DA, Edwards-George J, Dennis M, et al. Factors that influence adherence to a gluten-free diet in adults with celiac disease. Dig Dis Sci 2008;53(6): 1573–81.
73. O'Leary C, Wieneke P, Healy M, et al. Celiac disease and the transition from childhood to adulthood: a 28-year follow-up. Am J Gastroenterol 2004;99(12): 2437–41.
74. O'Mahony S, Howdle PD, Losowsky MS. Review article: management of patients with non-responsive coeliac disease. Aliment Pharmacol Ther 1996;10(5): 671–80.
75. Stewart M, Andrews CN, Urbanski S, et al. The association of coeliac disease and microscopic colitis: a large population-based study. Aliment Pharmacol Ther 2011;33(12):1340–9.
76. Williams JJ, Kaplan GG, Makhija S, et al. Microscopic colitis-defining incidence rates and risk factors: a population-based study. Clin Gastroenterol Hepatol 2008;6(1):35–40.
77. Leeds JS, Höroldt BS, Sidhu R, et al. Is there an association between coeliac disease and inflammatory bowel diseases? A study of relative prevalence in comparison with population controls. Scand J Gastroenterol 2007;42(10):1214–20.
78. Rabsztyn A, Green PH, Berti I, et al. Macroamylasemia in patients with celiac disease. Am J Gastroenterol 2001;96(4):1096–100.
79. O'Leary C, Wieneke P, Buckley S, et al. Celiac disease and irritable bowel-type symptoms. Am J Gastroenterol 2002;97(6):1463–7.
80. Midhagen G, Hallert C. High rate of gastrointestinal symptoms in celiac patients living on a gluten-free diet: controlled study. Am J Gastroenterol 2003;98(9): 2023–6.
81. Richey R, Howdle P, Shaw E, et al. Recognition and assessment of coeliac disease in children and adults: summary of NICE guidance. BMJ 2009;338:b1684.
82. Chang MS, Minaya MT, Cheng J, et al. Double-blind randomized controlled trial of rifaximin for persistent symptoms in patients with celiac disease. Dig Dis Sci 2011;56(10):2939–46.
83. Corazza GR, Biagi F, Volta U, et al. Autoimmune enteropathy and villous atrophy in adults. Lancet 1997;350(9071):106–9.
84. Akram S, Murray JA, Pardi DS, et al. Adult autoimmune enteropathy: Mayo Clinic Rochester experience. Clin Gastroenterol Hepatol 2007;5(11):1282–90 [quiz: 1245].

85. Inagaki-Ohara K, Chinen T, Matsuzaki G, et al. Mucosal T cells bearing TCRgammadelta play a protective role in intestinal inflammation. J Immunol 2004;173(2): 1390–8.

86. Al-Toma A, Verbeek WH, Hadithi M, et al. Survival in refractory coeliac disease and enteropathy-associated T-cell lymphoma: retrospective evaluation of single-centre experience. Gut 2007;56(10):1373–8.

87. Rubio-Tapia A, Murray JA. Classification and management of refractory coeliac disease. Gut 2010;59(4):547–57.

88. Meijer JW, Mulder CJ, Goerres MG, et al. Coeliac disease and (extra)intestinal T-cell lymphomas: definition, diagnosis and treatment. Scand J Gastroenterol Suppl 2004;(241):78–84.

89. Goerres MS, Meijer JW, Wahab PJ, et al. Azathioprine and prednisone combination therapy in refractory coeliac disease. Aliment Pharmacol Ther 2003;18(5): 487–94.

Diarrhea in Chronic Inflammatory Bowel Diseases

Heimo H. Wenzl, MD

KEYWORDS

- Ulcerative colitis • Crohn's disease • Microscopic colitis • Collagenous colitis
- Lymphocytic colitis • Infection • Resection

KEY POINTS

- About 80% of patients with inflammatory bowel diseases initially present with diarrhea.
- Defective fluid absorption by the inflamed bowel is the predominant pathophysiologic mechanism in many patients.
- Diarrhea may arise from a variety of conditions other than inflammation secondary to the disease.
- Careful assessment is required to allow treatment targeted at the underlying diarrheal mechanism(s).
- Uncritical interpretation of diarrhea as a consequence of inflammation caused by the disease can be detrimental and result in inadequate antiinflammatory therapy.

INTRODUCTION

Diarrhea is a prevalent symptom and sign of patients with inflammatory bowel diseases (IBDs) and affects most patients. It may represent the first perceived manifestation of intestinal inflammation that brings these patients to the attention of physicians and remain a relevant problem throughout the course of the disease. In a recent population-based study,[1] 77% of patients with ulcerative colitis and 82% of patients with Crohn's disease (CD) presented with diarrhea at onset of disease. In the microscopic colitis syndrome, diarrhea is present by definition.[2] The severity of diarrhea in IBDs varies widely. Some patients pass slightly increased numbers of soft stools without major impact on activities of everyday life; for them, the symptoms may be merely an annoying nuisance. On the other end of the spectrum, the diarrhea can be so severe that substitution of water and electrolytes is required to compensate for enteral losses. More often, the diarrhea is not voluminous but it is persistent and

The author has nothing to disclose.
Division of Gastroenterology and Hepatology, Department of Internal Medicine, Medical University of Graz, Auenbruggerplatz 15, 8036 Graz, Austria
E-mail address: heimo.wenzl@klinikum-graz.at

Gastroenterol Clin N Am 41 (2012) 651–675
http://dx.doi.org/10.1016/j.gtc.2012.06.006
0889-8553/12/$ – see front matter © 2012 Elsevier Inc. All rights reserved.

associated with incapacitating and socially devastating urgency and fecal incontinence. In the typical patient, the diarrhea is intermittent, waxing and waning depending on the inflammatory activity of the disease.

Because diarrhea is so common and its severity is related to the intensity and extent of bowel inflammation, it is widely used as an index of disease activity and therapeutic response. Symptoms and signs pertaining to diarrhea (above all, stool frequency) are invariably present in scoring systems that gauge the clinical activity of IBDs. However, not all diarrhea is secondary to activated bowel inflammation. Particularly in patients with CD, conditions such as malabsorption of bile acids, fat, or carbohydrates, infection with *Clostridium difficile*, fistulas, a lack of absorptive surface because of previous resection, bacterial overgrowth or other causes may prevail, or add to the diarrhea caused by the disease per se. Moreover, defective function of the anal sphincter apparatus may aggravate symptoms and further complicate the clinical situation. Therefore, when a patient with IBD presents with diarrhea, careful assessment is warranted to define the causative mechanism(s) involved. Only then an individualized treatment plan can be tailored, targeting the pathophysiology relevant to the current problem. Uncritical interpretation of diarrhea as a consequence of inflammation caused by the disease can be detrimental because inadequate antiinflammatory therapy (eg, with steroids, or antibodies to tumor necrosis factor [TNF]) does not help and exposes patients to potentially dangerous side effects, and the unidentified cause of the problem (eg, an infective agent) is left untreated.

BRIEF REVIEW OF NORMAL INTESTINAL FLUID TRANSPORT

Before discussing diarrheal diseases, it may be useful to briefly review some principal issues concerning normal physiology of gastrointestinal fluid transport.

Normal people ingest about 2 L of fluid per day with food and drink, but 8 to 10 L enters the small intestine. The additional volume originates from digestive secretion that reaches the lumen in the form of saliva, gastric juice, bile, or pancreatic juice. Further fluid is constantly secreted from cells of the intestinal crypts. Most of the water is absorbed in the small intestine and about 600 to 1500 mL passes the ileocecal valve.[3] In the colon, almost all of the water that is not firmly bound to or associated with certain fecal solids (like undigested fiber and bacteria) is actively absorbed. Only 100 mL leaves the body with the stools. Thus, under normal conditions about 99% of the exogenous and endogenous fluid load is absorbed by the small bowel and the colon; if only 1 additional percent escapes absorption, excess water is likely to exist unbound to fecal solids, and stools become loose.[4] When more than 1500 mL/d is delivered from the small bowel into the cecum, the colon can increase absorption up to 4 to 6 L per day, but individual differences in the maximal absorptive capacity of the colon may be substantial. The critical load of fluid to the cecum also depends on entry rate, and diarrhea may sometimes result from a sudden increase of ileal flow. In healthy individuals, a 250-mL bolus of fluid rapidly delivered to the colon produced no symptoms, whereas a 500-mL bolus resulted in loose stools.[5]

MICROSCOPIC COLITIS
Background and Definition

The recognition of microscopic colitis as a cause of diarrhea is rather novel and the associated terminology has been confusing. Thirty-six years ago, Lindström[6] reported the case of a woman with chronic watery diarrhea and a grossly normal colon. Microscopy of rectal biopsy specimens revealed thick subepithelial collagenous deposits with plasmacytic infiltration in the lamina propria, and he named the condition collagenous colitis. Several years later, Read and colleagues[7] described a group of patients with a similar clinical picture and nonspecific mucosal inflammation without a thickened collagen layer; they coined the term microscopic colitis to denote the fact that colonic mucosa appears normal to the naked eye. Subsequently, the term lymphocytic colitis was introduced to point out that the presence of lymphocytes in the epithelium of the colonic mucosa is the hallmark histologic feature in these patients.[8] Currently, microscopic colitis is defined as a syndrome of watery diarrhea characterized by a normal colonoscopic appearance and histologic changes of lymphocytic-plasmacytic inflammation in the lamina propria and intraepithelial lymphocytosis, with or without thickening of the subepithelial collagen table.[9] If a thickened collagenous band is present beneath the surface epithelium, the term collagenous colitis is used; if there is no thickened band, the condition is categorized as lymphocytic colitis. Because clinical presentation, disease course, and response to therapy are so similar, collagenous colitis and lymphocytic colitis are widely considered to represent 2 histologic subtypes of microscopic colitis.

Epidemiology

Microscopic colitis was once believed to be a rare disorder, but is has now become evident that it is a common cause of chronic diarrhea. At a tertiary referral center, the diagnosis was established in 10% of patients with this problem.[10] In Olmsted county, 3.1 new cases per 100 000 inhabitants were recorded in 1 year for collagenous colitis and 5.5 for lymphocytic colitis, with a significant increase in the incidence of microscopic colitis over time.[11] Similar results have been reported from Canada[12] and Europe.[13] Most of the studies showed a predominance of females, especially for collagenous colitis. The peak age of onset is in the sixth and seventh decade of life, yet all ages (even children) may be affected. Increased awareness of microscopic colitis by clinicians and pathologists may have contributed to the observed increase in incidence rates.

Cause

The cause of microscopic colitis is unknown. According to 1 hypothesis, a hitherto undefined noxious agent of dietary or microbiologic origin triggers or causes a chronic inflammation of the colonic mucosa in susceptible individuals. This view is supported by the presence of increased numbers of T lymphocytes in the epithelial lining of the colonic epithelium, which could reflect an immunologic reaction to that agent. In addition, when the fecal stream of patients with refractory collagenous colitis was diverted by an ileostomy, diarrhea ceased and the thickened subepithelial collagenous layer became normal.[14] Clinical symptoms and the abnormal collagen layer recurred after restoration of intestinal continuity. Many patients with microscopic colitis also have autoimmune or rheumatologic diseases, further supporting involvement of the immune system. Microscopic colitis has also been related to the ingestion of different drugs, including aspirin, nonsteroidal antiinflammatory drugs (NSAIDs), proton pump inhibitors, ranitidine, sertraline, ticlopidine, acarbose, flutamide, and simvastatin.[15] In some patients, withdrawal of the incriminated drug can lead to resolution of symptoms; in others, drug-induced diarrhea may have uncovered preexistent microscopic colitis. A further intraluminal factor is gluten. There exists a link between microscopic colitis and celiac sprue, with the concomitance of the 2 diseases being 50 times higher than expected in the general population[16]; 5.2% to 9% of patients with microscopic colitis also have celiac sprue.[16–19] Several HLA-DQ loci have been identified to be linked with the occurrence of both microscopic colitis and celiac sprue,[20] which suggests the possibility that similar immune mechanisms are involved.[21] However, it is unlikely that gluten is the trigger of microscopic colitis.[20,21]

Pathophysiology of Diarrhea

In vivo perfusion studies revealed that colonic ion transport is substantially impaired in patients with lymphocytic colitis and collagenous colitis.[22,23] The predominant abnormality is a reduction of active and passive absorption of sodium and chloride, resulting in markedly depressed fluid absorption from the lumen of the colon.[22] Recent in vitro experiments performed on colonic biopsy specimens from patients with collagenous colitis also showed reduced sodium and chloride absorption to be the main diarrheal mechanisms accompanied by altered diffusion and downregulation of tight junction molecules.[24] Colonic fluid absorption and stool volume are dependent on the cellularity of the lamina propria[25] but not on collagen table thickening[26]; the more inflammatory cells are present in the lamina propria, the less water and electrolytes are absorbed and the higher is the volume of diarrheal stools. These findings are most consistent with inflammation-driven genesis of diarrhea. Although not studied in detail in this setting, it is conceivable that abnormal ion transport is a consequence of the presence of increased local cytokines and other mediators released by the inflammatory process. Because colonic absorption is severely depressed and net secretion is not frequently noted,[22] daily stool volume in microscopic colitis usually does not exceed the volume of fluid entering the colon each day (approximately 1000 mL) and averages about 500 mL.[2,27] Stool volumes greater than 1000 mL/d or the presence of steatorrhea usually indicate the coexistence of celiac sprue.[2]

In addition to inflammation, malabsorption of bile acids may also be present[28,29] and aggravate diarrhea in some patients with collagenous colitis. However, bile acid malabsorption has been observed in many other diarrheal diseases[30] and is an unlikely cause or main pathophysiologic mechanism of collagenous colitis.[21] Treatment with bile acid–binding resins resulted in rapid symptomatic improvement in many of these patients but also in patients without bile acid wasting.[28]

CLINICAL PRESENTATION

Chronic watery diarrhea is the main symptom in patients with microscopic colitis. Passage of blood, pus, or excess fat is atypical; in these situations, other causes should be sought. Severe abdominal pain and abdominal tenderness are also atypical, whereas cramping and abdominal discomfort associated with diarrhea are not unusual. Onset of symptoms can be insidious or sudden.[17,18,31] When diarrhea abruptly occurs, it may suggest an infectious process, but microbiological evaluation of the stool remains negative. Daily stool weight typically amounts to 300 to 700 g, and may exceed 1500 g in severe cases.[7,27,32] Dehydration is rare and the need for intravenous fluid substitution is exceptional. Stool frequency usually ranges between 3 and 10 bowel movements per day.[31–34] Stools are watery or runny in 23% to 70% of patients[31,32,35]; the rest have decreased fecal consistency of various degrees, depending on diet and other factors. Many have nocturnal diarrhea. Urgency is often present and 9% to 60 % of patients suffer from fecal incontinence.[18,19,33,34] Incontinence may be favored because the disease is more common in elderly women, in whom incontinence is also more prevalent. However, in a recent study, collagenous colitis was not associated with rectal hypersensitivity or disturbed anal function.[36] On the contrary, when a balloon was distended in the inflamed rectum of these patients, they had a higher rectal pressure threshold and rectal volume at the feeling of first sensation.[36] This finding is different from findings in patients with active ulcerative colitis, who typically have reduced rectal compliance.

Because these symptoms are nonspecific, they may erroneously be attributed to diarrhea-predominant irritable bowel syndrome (IBS), especially in younger women with mild disease. Other causes of watery diarrhea are listed in **Box 1**.

DIAGNOSIS

Diagnosis of microscopic colitis is usually straightforward, provided it is considered as a differential diagnosis. Because recognition of both lymphocytic and collagenous colitis is based entirely on histologic examination of colonic mucosa, it is essential that in patients presenting with chronic watery diarrhea, multiple biopsies (six to ten) are taken from different parts of the apparently normal colon. In most instances, the correct diagnosis can be established by initial use of sigmoidoscopy.[10,37] Occasionally, initial samples are nondiagnostic as a result of discontinuous or patchy distribution of disease[38]; in this situation, full colonoscopy with biopsies taken from both the right and the left side of the colon should be performed.[39,40] Depending on the clinical situation, colonoscopy is frequently performed initially to avoid false-negative results or to rule out other potential causes of the patient's symptoms or coexisting carcinoma. It is also important that biopsy specimens are interpreted by a skilled pathologist who has been provided with information relevant to the case.

TREATMENT OF MICROSCOPIC COLITIS

Medical treatment options for microscopic colitis were analyzed in a recent Cochrane review.[41] The results showed budesonide to be an effective treatment, and suggested that bismuth subsalicylate, prednisone, and mesalamine with or without cholestyramine may be beneficial.[41] As an initial step in management of patients, NSAIDs and any other agents or dietary factors that might aggravate symptoms should be discontinued if possible; specific dietary recommendation or management is not available. To test for concurrent celiac sprue, serologic studies (tissue transglutaminase with an IgA level) can be performed. In patients with severe diarrhea, steatorrhea significant weight loss, unexplained iron deficiency anemia, or other signs of celiac disease, as well as in patients who are refractory to medical therapy, duodenal biopsies should be obtained.

Nonspecific Antidiarrheal Drugs

Antimotility medications, such as loperamide, are commonly prescribed first and often give satisfactory control of diarrhea in mild cases. In retrospective studies, a response was observed in 50% to 70% of patients.[17–19] Resolution of diarrhea was less common (13%–23%).[19,33]

Budesonide

Budesonide is the most thoroughly studied drug in the treatment of patients with microscopic colitis. Budesonide (9 mg/d) induces clinical and histologic response in both lymphocytic colitis and collagenous colitis, and maintains responses in collagenous colitis.[41] Analysis of pooled data from controlled trials shows that after 6 to 8 weeks of treatment, a clinical response was noted in 81% of patients with collagenous colitis (placebo 17%) and in 86% of patients with lymphocytic colitis (placebo 40%).[41] In collagenous colitis, continued treatment with budesonide at a lower dose (6 mg/d) could maintain response for 6 months in 75% of initial responders to induction therapy with 9 mg/d (placebo 25%).[41] Discontinuation of therapy is frequently followed by

Box 1
Differential diagnosis of chronic watery diarrhea

Microscopic colitis

Malabsorption of carbohydrates and sugar alcohols

    Lactose, fructose

    Sorbitol

Laxative abuse

    Magnesium, sulfate, phosphate, lactulose

    Senna, bisacodyl, phenolphthalein, ricinoleic acid

Endocrine diarrhea

    Diabetic diarrhea

    Thyroid disease

    Addison disease

Bile acid diarrhea

Amyloidosis

Mast cell disease

Small bowel bacterial overgrowth

Mesenteric ischemia

Iatrogenic diarrhea

    Drugs

    Postresection diarrhea

    Radiation enteritis

    Postvagotomy, postsympathectomy

Epidemic secretory diarrhea

Idiopathic secretory diarrhea

Poisons

Neoplasia

    Colon carcinoma

    Lymphoma

    Villous adenoma

IBS

Giardiasis

Collagen-vascular diseases

Tuberculosis

Circulating secretagogues

    Gastrin

    Vasoactive intestinal polypeptide

    Calcitonin

    Somatostatin

    Glucagon

    Serotonin

    Histamine

Lymphangiectasia

Ulcerative colitis

CD

relapse, but symptoms usually respond to reintroduction of budesonide. Many patients maintain remission on lower doses (3–6 mg/d). Patients on long-term therapy with budesonide need to be monitored for steroid side effects. Budesonide is considered the drug of first choice in patients with moderate to severe symptoms, or when symptoms persist despite other therapy.

Bismuth Subsalicylate

Bismuth subsalicylate has antiinflammatory and antibacterial effects. In 1 study, 90% of patients with microscopic colitis reached a clinical remission; in 80%, histologic improvement was noted.[32] Similar results were obtained in a small controlled trial.[42] Patients daily ingested 9 tablets of bismuth subsalicylate (262 mg each) in 3 divided doses. Response to bismuth subsalicylate usually occurs within 1 month of continuous treatment. In responders, the drug is usually given for a second month. Remission may last more than 2 years.[32] Because bismuth subsalicylate is inexpensive and well tolerated, it can be tried initially in patients with mild or moderate diarrhea. In many countries, bismuth subsalicylate is not available because of concerns regarding long-term toxicity.

Cholestyramine

This anion-binding resin may alleviate diarrhea in patients with microscopic colitis with or without bile acid malabsorption. It has been speculated that the resin binds to an unknown offending agent that stimulates the inflammatory process. There have been several clinical observations,[17–19] open-label studies,[28,43] and 1 controlled trial[44] suggesting clinical efficacy without constant improvement of inflammatory histology. The effective dose required for satisfactory control of diarrhea varies between patients (2–24 g/d), but most of those who respond need 4 to 12 g/d (1–3 packages of cholestyramine).[28,43] Because of its taste and texture, it is difficult for many patients to ingest cholestyramine over longer periods. Nevertheless, cholestyramine may be helpful in patients with mild or moderate diarrhea and is an option in those resistant to steroid therapy.

5-Aminosalicylate Drugs

5-Aminosalicylate drugs have frequently been used in patients with microscopic colitis. In 1 unblinded study without placebo control, patients ingested mesalazine 800 mg 3 times daily alone or in combination with 4 g of cholestyramine for 6 months.[44] Clinical and histologic remission reportedly occurred in 85% of patients with lymphocytic colitis and in 91% of patients with collagenous colitis, the latter benefitting more from additional cholestyramine.[44] In uncontrolled series, a response was noted in less than half of the patients.[17,18] Preliminary data from a randomized trial indicate that mesalazine is ineffective in collagenous colitis.[45] At interim analysis clinical remission at 8 weeks was observed in 44% of patients treated with 3 g mesalazine granules; remission rates for placebo and budesonide (9 mg) were 59.5% and 80%, respectively.

Prednisolone

One small placebo-controlled trial showed a trend toward improvement in stool frequency[46] after treatment with prednisolone 50 mg for 2 weeks. Systemic steroids are an option when budesonide fails, but responders are likely to relapse after discontinuation of therapy.

Azathioprine, 6-Mercaptopurine, and Methotrexate

These immunosuppressive drugs may be beneficial in steroid refractory or dependent patients.[47] In 1 retrospective analysis of patients with collagenous colitis, treatment with methotrexate was followed by clinical improvement of symptoms in 16 of

19 cases.[48] The median methotrexate dose was 7.5–10 mg and the dose range was 5–25 mg orally once a week.

Anti-TNF Drugs

According to recent small case series[49,50] treatment with TNF-blockers (infliximab and adalimumab) was highly effective in inducing clinical remission in patients with refractory severe lymphocytic and collagenous colitis. In 1 study[49] long term clinical remission (more than 1 year) was achieved in 3 of 4 patients. More data is required to define the role of anti-TNF therapy in this setting. The potential benefit of systemic steroids, immunosuppressives and anti-TNF drugs has to be weighed against the risks of drug-induced complications in the often elderly patients.

Most patients respond sufficiently to medical management. Surgery (ileostomy, with or without colectomy, or colectomy with ileal pouch-anal anastomosis) is reserved for those rare patients with debilitating diarrhea in whom all forms of medical therapy have been exhausted without success.[14,19,51]

ULCERATIVE COLITIS AND CD

Different from microscopic colitis, that has been considered a gentler and more subtle form of colitis,[52] the classic IBDs (ulcerative colitis and CD) are characterized by more severe, macroscopically visible, inflammatory changes in the gut that usually entail destruction of the mucosal surface, with structures beyond the mucosa also being affected in CD. These 2 illnesses are more serious; they can be life-threatening and are associated with an increased risk of colorectal carcinoma.

Ulcerative colitis is a diffuse inflammation that primarily affects the colonic mucosa. It almost always involves the rectum and may extend proximally in a continuous fashion along a variable length of the colon. At initial presentation, disease is limited to the rectum in 30%, and does not reach beyond the splenic flexure in two-thirds of patients.[1] In more than half of the patients, inflammation progresses with time to involve more proximal parts of the colon. Thus, topical therapy that reaches only distal parts of the colon may become inefficient in a patient with proximal progression of disease. The small bowel is not affected, with the exception of slight inflammation of the terminal ileum, which is referred to as backwash ileitis.

CD can involve any segment of the intestinal tube, from the mouth to the anus. Typically, the distal small bowel and the proximal colon are affected. About 25% of patients have colonic involvement only, and in about one-third of cases only the small intestine is inflamed. Distribution of inflammatory lesions is patchy and discontinuous, with normal-appearing segments of the intestine between affected areas. The behavior of CD can be inflammatory, stricturing, or penetrating, with progression to the penetrating variant with time.

CLINICAL PRESENTATION

Patients with ulcerative colitis present with a variable spectrum of symptoms and signs that are largely determined by the anatomic extent and intensity of inflammation in the colon.[53] When the disease is limited to the rectum or rectosigmoid, recurrent or persistent rectal bleeding associated with the passage of mucus and small loose stools is common. In most patients with active disease, the number of bowel movements is increased. When the rectum is inflamed, many patients lose the ability to discriminate fecal matter from gas and experience a feeling of incomplete evacuation. Rectal compliance may be restricted, so that stool cannot be sufficiently withheld, and patients may be distressed by urgent defecation and incontinence. With more proximal extension of disease, diarrhea tends to become more severe and patients may pass more than 10 bloody stools per day. Abdominal cramps are often associated with the diarrhea. Nocturnal and postprandial diarrhea is common.

In CD, diarrhea is highly variable depending on gut segments affected and the diarrheal mechanisms involved. Patients with disease limited to the colon may have symptoms similar to patients with ulcerative colitis. When the small and the large intestine are inflamed, stool volume can be high because the diseased colon cannot fully compensate for increased fluid volumes delivered from the small intestine.

Not all patients with ulcerative colitis or CD present with diarrhea. One-third of patients with active proctitis or proctosigmoiditis may void pellets of hard stools.[53] In CD, about 20% of patients initially present without diarrhea[1]; other symptoms, such as right lower abdominal pain or arthralgias, may dominate the clinical picture. Diarrhea often develops later, for example as a consequence of bowel resection.

PATHOPHYSIOLOGY OF DIARRHEA

The pathophysiology of diarrhea in IBD is multifactorial and complex. Inflammation clearly is the most important factor that finally results in abnormal intestinal ion transport and motor function. However, a variety of noninflammatory mechanisms may coexist, or precipitate diarrhea in the absence of inflammation.

INFLAMMATION AND DEFECTIVE INTESTINAL ION TRANSPORT

In ulcerative colitis, the principal disturbance that leads to the development of diarrhea is a profound decrease in the net absorption of sodium (and consequently of chloride and water) from the lumen of the colon.[54,55] The failure to absorb salt and water is considered primarily a consequence of reduced activity of the Na+/K+-adenosine triphosphatase (ATPase) pump located in the basolateral membrane of colonocytes[56–58] and of an impaired function of apical sodium channels.[59–61] These channels are present in surface colonocytes located in the distal large bowel, where ulcerative colitis is invariably present. In addition, the epithelial barrier may be leaky because of apoptotic foci[62] and altered tight junction structure,[63] which is supposed to favor back leakage of absorbed fluid across the tight junctions into the lumen. By contrast, excessive active anion secretion, which is the underlying basis of several infectious diarrheal diseases (eg, cholera, enterotoxic *Escherichia coli*) and of diarrhea caused by endogenous secretagogues (eg, vasoactive intestinal peptide[64]), does not seem to have major importance.[65] This finding is in line with the observation that patients with the large bowel uncoupled by ileostomy do not have much discharge from the isolated colon, even although it may remain intensely inflamed.[66]

Reduced net absorption of salt and water is also present in patients with CD of the large[67] and small bowel.[68] In addition to defective sodium absorption,[57,69,70] active secretion may be important in the generation of diarrhea[71] in some patients. Sodium transport has recently been shown to be reduced in colonocytes from the macroscopically noninflamed bowel of patients with small intestinal CD.[72] Abnormal function of macroscopically normal intestine has also been noted in early perfusion studies, in which reduced sodium flux was detected in the radiologically normal small intestine of colectomized patients with CD.[68] Thus, fluid absorption can be disturbed in areas of the intestine with an apparently normal morphology.

The changes in ion transport, as described earlier, are primarily a consequence of inflammation. A multitude of immune and inflammatory mediators are present in the intestinal mucosa of patients with IBD and are likely to alter colonocyte function and bowel motility directly or via endocrine cells and elements of the enteric nervous system. In experimental animals, proinflammatory cytokines such as TNF-α and interferon γ have been shown to impair the expression of sodium channels, reduce epithelial Na+/K+-ATPase activity, and increase mucosal permeability,[73,74] leading to decreased intestinal sodium and water absorption. Therapeutic blockade of proinflammatory cytokines (eg, with antibodies to TNF) can reverse these effects and improve diarrhea in patients with IBD.

Inflammation also causes denudation of the epithelium, favoring leakage of plasmalike fluid and blood into the lumen, augmenting intestinal fluid load. In addition, the absorptive surface may be diminished because of ulcers. In some patients, the failure of the inflamed colon to salvage unabsorbed carbohydrates may have a role.[75,76]

Diarrhea can also be accentuated by disturbances of intestinal motility.[77] Although diarrhea in general goes along with accelerated intestinal transit, motor abnormalities may not be uniform but rather vary between segments of the gut. For example, many patients with active ulcerative colitis have proximal colonic stasis, whereas transit through the rectosigmoid region is rapid.[78] Therefore, antidiarrheal drugs that further slow proximal colonic transit should be used with caution in these patients.[78] The distal colon seems to be programmed to react to intraluminal contents by generating strong contractions that challenge the continence mechanism and cause frequent, urgent, and often painful defecation.[79] In patients with CD, intestinal obstruction can impede normal flow of intestinal contents and cause diarrhea as a consequence of bacterial overgrowth (see later discussion).

CAUSES OF DIARRHEA OTHER THAN INFLAMMATION RESULTING FROM ACTIVE DISEASE

Not all diarrhea in patients with IBD originates from active inflammation caused by the disease. Especially in CD, a wide variety of potential mechanisms can interfere with normal absorption of nutrients and fluid. It is important to understand the pathophysiologic basis of these mechanisms to better identify the cause or causes responsible for the diarrhea in an individual patient (**Table 1**).

Malabsorption

Diarrhea can result from malabsorption of bile acids, fat, and carbohydrate.

Bile acids are produced in the liver and secreted as conjugates of glycin or taurine into bile. After a fatty meal the gallbladder contracts and bile acids enter the small intestine, where they assist fat absorption. Bile acids are avidly reabsorbed by the terminal ileum and are then returned to the liver via the portal blood. This continuous cycle of secretion, absorption, and resecretion is termed the enterohepatic circulation.[80] With each meal, the bile acid pool, which weighs about 2 to 3 g in adults, cycles several times. Under normal conditions, ileal reabsorption of bile acids is highly efficient: less than 5% of bile acids secreted enter the colon and are excreted in feces. When the terminal ileum is severely inflamed, resected, or bypassed by a fistula, more bile acids escape absorption and reach the colon. Here, dihydroxy bile acids inhibit water and electrolyte absorption and stimulate fluid secretion, resulting in diarrhea. Sequestration of bile acids by binding resins can lessen the diarrhea.[81,82] Bile acid losses are compensated by increased hepatic synthesis, providing bile acid concentrations in the small intestinal chyme high enough to enable micelle formation and adequate lipid absorption. This situation is often present when less than 50 cm of the terminal ileum is missing. If there is extensive ileal resection (about >100 cm) bile acid losses begin to exceed hepatic synthesis and micelle formation becomes insufficient. Excess fat reaches the colon,[83] where bacteria transform long-chain fatty acids

Table 1
Approach to patients with IBD and diarrhea

Cause	Diagnostic Approaches	Treatment
Inflammation caused by IBD	Blood chemistry Stool markers Endoscopy Radiologic imaging studies	Antiinflammatory medication Immunosuppressives Biologicals
Enteric infection	History of recent antibiotic therapy or previous infection with *Clostridium difficile* Microbiological stool tests Colonoscopy + biopsy (cytomegalovirus?)	Antimicrobial therapy
Malabsorption	Dietary history Breath tests Stool analyses [^{75}Se]Selena-homocholic acid conjugated with taurine, diagnostic trial with cholestyramine	Bile acids: binding resins Fat: low-fat diet, bile acid replacement Carbohydrate: avoid lactose and fructose
Bacterial overgrowth	Presence of predisposing abnormalities Bacterial culture from jejunal aspirate Breath tests	Antibiotics Dilatation of strictures Surgery
Postresection	Review of surgical history Radiologic imaging Endoscopy	Antidiarrheal medication Stool modifiers Frequent feedings, avoid caffeine Histamine$_2$-receptor blockers, proton pump inhibitors Replacement of fluid and nutrients
Fistula	History of halitosis or fecal vomiting Radiologic imaging Endoscopy	Surgery
Medication	History	Discontinue offending agent
Food intolerance	History	Avoid offending diet
IBS	History Endoscopy, radiologic imaging and additional tests as required to exclude other causes	Fiber supplements Antispasmodics, antidiarrheal agents Tricyclic antidepressants

to hydroxylated fatty acids (molecules resembling ricinoleic acid), which elicit fluid secretion in the colon and diarrhea. Because water malabsorption in the small intestine dilutes bile acid concentration in the colon less than the cathartic threshold of 3 to 5 mmol/L,[84] bile acid–induced fluid secretion in the large bowel does not contribute importantly to the diarrhea. In this situation, binding resins do not work, but a low-fat diet may ameliorate the steatorrhea.[85] Because the bile acid pool becomes progressively depleted during the day, high-fat loads should be avoided, particularly in the evening. In some patients with extensive bowel resection, bile acid deficiency, and steatorrhea, fat absorption could be improved by supplementation with exogenous bile acid,[86–88] but availability may be a problem.

Steatorrhea can occur in patients with CD also by mechanisms other than bile acid deficiency (eg, because of limited absorptive surface area or small intestinal bacterial overgrowth [see later discussion]).

Diarrhea in patients with CD can also be associated with malabsorption of carbohydrate.[89] Most of the ~275 g of carbohydrate that normal people eat per day[90] is absorbed in the upper small intestine; 25 g may reach the colon physiologically.[91] If there is extensive small intestinal inflammation or resection, increased amounts of carbohydrate may enter the colon. In the colon where bacterial fermentation generates short-chain fatty acids that are partly absorbed; the unabsorbed molecules (organic anions and carbohydrate) cause osmotic diarrhea.[89] Bacterial fermentation of carbohydrate also generates gas, which may give rise to abdominal distension, pain, and excess flatus. Whether or not diarrhea occurs after ingestion of a particular carbohydrate depends (in addition to the capacity of digestive and absorptive mechanisms in the small intestine) on the mass, the capacity of colonic bacteria to metabolize unabsorbed carbohydrate, and the capacity of the colonic mucosa to absorb the products of bacterial metabolism.[91,92] Severe malabsorption of carbohydrate has been noted after resectional surgery of both the large and the small bowel.[89]

Malabsorption of lactose is often diagnosed in patients with IBD[93–96] and its prevalence primarily depends on the frequency of primary lactose malabsorption in the background population. Although the issue is controversial, lactose malabsorption seems to be more prevalent in patients with CD than in normal controls,[93,95] particularly when the small bowel is affected.[95] However, a varying fraction of these patients remain asymptomatic when they malabsorb lactose or ingest milk. For example, in 1 study, 11 patients malabsorbed lactose after ingestion of 250 mL milk, but only 3 of them experienced symptoms of intolerance.[93] In another study, 19 of 21 patients with a positive lactose breath test also reported symptoms after milk ingestion; milk intolerance was reported by 83% of patients with active CD, but could not be sufficiently explained by lactase levels in the duodenal mucosa.[96] Apart from primary or secondary reduction of hydrolase activity in the brush border membrane, malabsorption of sugar may also arise from other factors such as bacterial overgrowth and increased intestinal motility. Patients may become intolerant to lactose only after they have developed IBD; therefore a normal lactose breath test before the onset of IBD does not exclude current lactose malabsorption.

Diagnosis of lactose malabsorption is usually confirmed by lactose hydrogen breath test. Upper endoscopy with duodenal biopsies is suitable to investigate the mucosa for inflammatory changes caused by the disease and to rule out celiac disease, which may also cause secondary lactose malabsorption. Stool tests may also be helpful, because a low fecal pH is characteristic for diarrhea caused by carbohydrate malabsorption. A fecal pH less than 5.3 indicates that carbohydrate malabsorption is a major cause of diarrhea, whereas a pH greater than 5.6 argues against carbohydrate malabsorption as the only cause of diarrhea.[37,97]

Lactose restriction frequently ameliorates symptoms but diarrhea usually does not subside completely, presumably because additional mechanisms remain active. In secondary lactase deficiency caused by inflammatory changes, antiinflammatory therapy may restore lactase function.

Fistulas and Bacterial Overgrowth

Patients with CD may develop fistulas between different loops of bowel. As a consequence, intraluminal content may bypass a sizable length of the gut and cause diarrhea. Ileosigmoid fistulas are the most common type of fistula between 2 loops of bowel and occur in up to 6% of patients with CD.[98,99] Gastrocolic fistulas are less frequent and may present with halitosis and fecal vomiting.

Another condition that may cause diarrhea and mimic an acute flare of CD is small bowel bacterial overgrowth.[100] In contrast to the colon, which harbors a very large microbiota, the small bowel is sparsely populated with bacteria. This low concentration of bacteria is maintained by the cleansing action of antegrade peristalsis and an intact ileocecal valve that restricts reflux of cecal contents into the ileum. If the regular flow of small intestinal content is disturbed, bacteria tend to overgrow intestinal segments where stasis occurred, leading to diarrhea, steatorrhea, malabsorption, and weight loss. Bacteria may provoke diarrhea by the release of toxins that act on the intestinal mucosa and by deconjugation of conjugated bile acids to deconjugated bile acids. As a consequence, fewer conjugated bile acids are available in the small intestine to assist fat absorption and steatorrhea may result. Deconjugated bile acids can be toxic to the mucosa and disrupt the epithelial surface; they are rapidly absorbed in the jejunum.

In patients with CD, several anatomic abnormalities that predispose to overgrowth of bacteria are frequently present.[101–103] Strictures can cause stagnation of intraluminal content, and internal fistulas may leave segments of the small bowel out of continuity with the regular flow or provide an abnormal connection between the colon and the small bowel or the stomach. Bacterial counts in the distal small intestine may also be abnormally increased when the ileocecal valve has been resected or rendered incompetent by disease. When patients with CD were studied using breath tests, bacterial overgrowth was more common after ileocecal resection and other resective procedures[100,103] as well as in patients with intestinal strictures,[102] and was related to bloating and diarrhea.[100]

Direct confirmation of bacterial overgrowth can be obtained only by qualitative and quantitative culture of fluid aspirated from the upper small bowel ($>10^6$ bacteria/mL). Indirect tests include the 14C-D-xylose breath test, the 14C-glycocholate breath test, and the hydrogen breath tests with lactulose or glucose. The latter are more frequently used than invasive aspirate culture, but interpretation of respective results may be difficult because of limited sensitivity and specificity, especially in the presence of diarrhea. Thus, it may be difficult to determine the extent to which diarrhea is attributable to overgrowth of bacteria. If specific tests are not available or test results are inconclusive, empiric therapy is often instituted in the presence of anatomic abnormalities that might favor stasis.

Postresection Diarrhea

Most patients with CD undergo resective surgery during the course of the disease, and not few require more than 1 operation. In the typical situation, the terminal ileum, the ileocecal valve, and part of the right colon are removed. After this type of operation, many (but not all) patients have diarrhea of varying severity. Pathophysiologic mechanisms involved include a reduction of absorptive surface specialized to absorb sodium against concentration gradients, loss of the gatekeeper function of the ileocecal valve, and loss of the ileal break (under normal conditions, entry of excess nutrients into the ileum decreases transit in more proximal sections of the intestine). Thus, an excessive load of unabsorbed fluid may flush the remaining colon and overwhelm its absorptive capacity. Malabsorbed bile acids and fats can induce colonic secretion and further aggravate diarrhea (see earlier discussion).

Diarrhea can also be a relevant problem after numerous other resective procedures performed in patients with IBD, such as proctocolectomy with ileoanal anastomosis, ileoanal pouch procedures, or permanent ileostomy.

A few patients with CD require such extensive intestinal resection that they develop short bowel syndrome. Loss of absorptive surface is the main pathophysiologic mechanism of diarrhea in these patients. Enhanced fluid secretion does also have a role, because diarrhea usually persists when patients fast. Secretion in the upper intestine is supposed to be high because antisecretory factors that would normally be released from the distal small bowel are lacking after resection. Malabsorption of nutrients can be substantial and further augment fecal output. Parenteral substitution of water and electrolytes may be necessary in these patients.

For appropriate assessment of postresection diarrhea, exact knowledge of the anatomic situation is pivotal. Therefore, all surgical records should be reviewed to estimate the length of intestinal sections still in situ. If this information is not available, endoscopic or radiologic evaluation may be necessary.

Many patients with intestinal resection have mild diarrhea (eg, 3–5 loose stools per day) in the absence of inflammation and often consider their bowel habits as being normal. Others have more pronounced diarrhea and may require nonspecific antidiarrheal treatment. However, it is important not to misinterpret this diarrhea as a consequence of increased disease activity, because antiinflammatory measures are not effective (with the possible exception of cortisone, which has an unspecific antidiarrheal effect). By the same token, antiinflammatory therapy for an inflammatory flare caused by the disease should not be considered ineffective in such patients when diarrhea does not resolve (but remits to the baseline level).

Infectious Causes

A further cause of diarrheal relapse in patients with IBD is enteric infection.[104] A wide variety of pathogenic micro-organisms have been reported in association with relapse of IBD, of which *Clostridium difficile* was most common. In 1 retrospective study from the United Kingdom, about 10% of relapses were associated with infections, of which 5.5% were caused by *Clostridium difficile* (the remainder was caused by a variety of other organisms like *Salmonella*, *Campylobacter*, *Entamoeba histolytica* and *Strongyloides*).[104] Most acquired *Clostridium difficile* as an outpatient and had been exposed to antibiotics. *Clostridium difficile*–associated disease (CDAD) of patients with IBD has recently increased in North America and is associated with a more severe course, greater likelihood of colectomy, and higher mortality than in patients with CDAD without underlying IBD.[105–107] Patients are particularly susceptible to CDAD when their IBD involves the colon. Endoscopically, the absence of pseudomembranes is common.[105] Clinicians need to be vigilant regarding this infection, especially in patients with active colitis, to identify the pathogen and start antibiotic therapy before embarking on immunosuppressive therapy.

Diarrhea in patients with IBD may result from any other intestinal infection that can occur in patients without IBD and produce clinical findings indistinguishable from an exacerbation of the disease. Therefore, microbiologic studies for bacterial infection (*Salmonella, Shigella, Yersinia, Campylobacter, Clostridium difficile, Escherichia coli 0157:H7*) and parasitic infestation should be considered in patients with known IBD who present with diarrhea, especially if they have had previous antibiotic therapy or infectious diarrhea, a relevant travel history, severe or refractory relapse, or when presenting symptoms differ from the patient-individual pattern of a diarrheal flare.[108–110]

Another clinical problem, which primarily arises in patients with severe colitis, is reactivation of cytomegalovirus infection (covered in the article on opportunistic infections by Krones and Högenauer elsewhere in this issue).

Side Effect of Medication

Diarrhea can be caused by medications used for treatment of IBD or associated problems. Aminosalicylates,[111,112] NSAIDs, antibiotics, iron pills, magnesium supplements, thiopurine drugs,[113,114] proton pump inhibitors, cholestyramine, and many other agents can induce or aggravate diarrhea by various mechanisms in susceptible patients. In occasional patients, drug-induced diarrhea can be severe.[112–114] It is important to obtain a detailed list of all drugs, remedies, and supplements that the patient used before onset of symptoms. Correlation with time identifies the offending agent in some patients, but often the causative role of medication become more evident only in retrospect.

IBS

A group of patients may present with symptoms similar to those reported by patients with IBS: they have intermittent cramping abdominal pain and diarrhea in the absence of inflammatory changes or other explanations for the severity of symptoms. The diagnosis of IBS is difficult to make in patients with IBD who have a chronic bowel disease that is incompletely understood, causes morphologic changes of the intestine, and extramural structures and frequently entails surgery. Nevertheless, IBS is common in the general population and should be considered as a complicating factor in patients with IBD.[115] Key to diagnosis is questioning patients about symptoms suggestive of IBS before the onset of their IBD.

Patient Assessment

History

The first step in assessing a patient with IBD and diarrhea is a thorough, detailed medical history. The history should include questions pertaining to the overall condition of the patient, changes in body weight, and the presence of systemic symptoms such as general weakness, fever, and night sweats. A history of low urine output may indicate volume depletion. Patients should also be questioned about the presence of extraintestinal symptoms including arthralgias, skin manifestations, eye manifestations, and aphthous ulcerations in the mouth. A detailed history should be obtained regarding bowel habits (ie, frequency and consistency of stools, patients' perception of stool volume) and associated symptoms such as abdominal pain, bloating, urgency, and incontinence. Characteristics of the stool itself, including the presence of visible blood, pus, mucus, fat, and undigested food particles may suggest a potential pathophysiologic mechanism and guide further evaluation. Patients rarely volunteer all of this information and need to be asked directly, in particular concerning incontinence. It is also important to review the diet history, with special attention to recent changes, because it may reveal lactose intolerance or exacerbation of symptoms after ingestion of fat, poorly absorbed sugars, or caffeine. All medications taken within the last 6 to 8 weeks should be recorded, and the temporal association of diarrhea with ingestion of drugs and other potentially prodiarrheic agents should be searched for.

Physical and Laboratory Examination

All patients with diarrhea require a physical examination. Attention should be given above all to signs of volume depletion and systemic inflammation. Therefore, evaluation of the hydration status, pulse, blood pressure, and body temperature is required. Inspection of the skin and the oral cavity may reveal erythema nodosum or aphthous ulcers. The abdomen should be examined to determine whether abdominal extension, tenderness, a palpable mass, or abnormal bowel sounds are present. Inspection of the anus may reveal fistula openings, fissures, or frank ulceration of the perianal skin; digital examination can give an impression of the anal sphincter pressure. To detect weight loss, patients should be weighed on a scale, because mere history of body weight may be incorrect.

Laboratory testing usually comprises a complete blood count and serum chemistries (including sodium, potassium, chloride, bicarbonate, creatinine, urea nitrogen, albumin, aspartate aminotransferase, alanine aminotransferase, alkaline phosphatase, and a C-reactive protein level). Measurement of serum micronutrients and vitamins, such as iron, magnesium, calcium, phosphorus, zinc, β-carotene, folic acid, and vitamin B_{12} are useful when malabsorption or specific deficiency states are suspected.

Microbial stool tests are necessary for detection of intestinal infection and should always be performed during refractory or severe relapse, and in those with a history of antibiotic therapy within an arbitrary 3 months.[116]

Analysis of the stool can provide important information. A spot sample is sufficient to test for the presence of occult blood, white blood cells (Wright stain, fecal lactoferrin, or fecal calprotectin assay) and fecal fat (Sudan stain) and thus to permit further classification of the diarrhea (watery, inflammatory, fatty). Quantitative stool collections for 48 or 72 hours provide a more accurate estimate of quantitative and qualitative fecal losses. Steatorrhea is present in a patient with diarrhea when fecal fat output exceeds 14 g per day.[117] Measurement of fecal electrolytes allows calculation of the fecal osmotic gap (290–2 × [fecal sodium concentration + fecal potassium concentration]); a value greater than 50 mOsm/kg points at an osmotic component to the diarrhea. A fecal pH less than 5.3 suggests that carbohydrate malabsorption is present.

As mentioned earlier, H2-breath tests with lactose or glucose and lactulose are useful when lactose malabsorption or bacterial overgrowth is suspected. The 14C-D-xylose breath test and the 14C-glycocholate breath test have also been used for assessment of bacterial overgrowth but are often not available.

Bile acid malabsorption can be measured by several laboratory tests, including those using ^{75}selena-homocholic acid conjugated with taurine[118] and ^{14}C-glycocholate. Because the specificity and availability of these methods is limited, many clinicians use a therapeutic trial of cholestyramine as an indirect test for the possibility that malabsorbed bile acids are the cause of diarrhea.[37]

Endoscopy and Imaging Studies

Ileocolonoscopy is appropriate to determine the extent and severity of inflammatory changes in the colon and terminal ileum. Other relevant abnormalities, such as stenosis or fistula openings, may also be visualized. However, the correlation between clinical symptoms and endoscopic disease activity is poor, especially in CD.[119] Therefore, the contribution of inflammation to the diarrhea may be difficult to estimate in some scenarios (eg, substantial diarrhea but only minor inflammatory changes in a patient with CD) and further assessment may be required.

Upper endoscopy is used in patients with CD to detect upper gastrointestinal involvement. Other causes of diarrhea, such as coexistent celiac disease, lambliasis, or small bowel bacterial overgrowth (aspiration of jejunal fluid) can also be diagnosed with the help of upper endoscopy.

Because CD may affect sections of bowel out of reach of a standard endoscope, radiologic imaging studies may be necessary. Fluoroscopic examinations are increasingly replaced by magnetic resonance (MR) imaging or computed tomography (CT) enterography/enteroclysis that have a higher sensitivity for the detection of small bowel lesions and can more accurately detect extraluminal complication. Because radiation exposure from fluoroscopy and CT is considerable, MR should be used when possible. In experienced hands, transabdominal ultrasonography may also be valuable for assessment of bowel inflammation and extraintestinal complications.

Small bowel capsule endoscopy (SBCE) is a novel method of directly visualizing small bowel lesions in patients with IBD that may be missed by traditional endoscopic or radiologic procedures.[120] In clinical practice, indications of SBCE are limited in patients with proven CD. It may be useful to determine the extent and severity of lesions in the small intestine, postoperative recurrence, and in the clinical setting of functional bowel disorders to assess whether inflammatory lesions are present.[120] Because partial bowel obstruction is frequent in CD and may cause capsule retention, it is prudent to perform small bowel imaging or to use a patency capsule (that disintegrates in case of retention) before SBCE.

TREATMENT

Before treatment is initiated, the putative mechanism(s) responsible for the diarrhea need to be defined. In most instances, exacerbation of diarrheal symptoms is the result of increased inflammatory activity of the disease. In this situation, control of inflammation is of foremost importance. Drugs directed at inducing and maintaining clinical remission include aminosalicylates, corticosteroids, immunosuppressives, and antibodies to TNF and adhesion molecules. Treatment algorithms have been developed and are constantly updated to guide clinicians in the use of these medications.[108,109,121,122]

In cases of enteric infection, appropriate antimicrobial therapy should be instituted. Mild to moderate *Clostridium difficile*–associated disease is initially treated with metronidazole.[123] The usual oral treatment regime is 200 to 250 mg 4 times daily or 400 to 500 mg 3 times daily for 10 to 14 days. Oral vancomycin is equally effective but more costly. In patients with symptoms of severe CDAD, or if the patient's condition fails to improve or deteriorates on metronidazole, then early use of vancomycin is recommended. Signs of severe CDAD include a systemic inflammatory response (tachycardia, fever), electrolyte imbalance, volume depletion, hypotension, ileus, toxic megacolon, or peritonitis. The dose of vancomycin for acute CDAD is 125 mg every 6 hours, which is of equivalent efficacy to 500 mg 4 times daily. Other antibiotics should be stopped if possible.[123]

If there is evidence of bacterial overgrowth antibiotics such as tetracyclines, trimethoprim/sulfamethoxazole, ciprofloxacin, metronidazole, or rifaximin can be considered. Specific literature on antibiotic treatment of bacterial overgrowth in CD is scarce. In 1 controlled study, ciprofloxacin (500 mg 2 times daily) as well as metronidazole (250 mg 3 times daily) was effective in this scenario.[124] Rifaximin (400 mg 3 times daily) had a transient effect without change of disease activity.[125] Antibiotics are usually prescribed for 7 to 10 days. As long as the predisposing anatomic abnormalities persist, repeated or periodic treatment courses may be necessary. In refractory cases, surgery may be necessary to abolish stasis.

In patients with ileal disease or resection, cholestyramine can ameliorate or abolish diarrhea by binding bile salts in the lumen of the intestine. Cholestyramine is given in divided doses before meals and separate from other medication. The optimal dose varies between patients and needs to be individually adapted according to efficacy and tolerability. Many patients do well on relatively small doses, for example, 2 g per day. Others may require higher quantities of cholestyramine (up to 16–24 g per day) to achieve the desired effect, but, at least in our experience, few take such high doses on a regular basis. If there is no improvement within a few days despite the patient ingesting a large dose, treatment can be stopped. In cases of intolerance to cholestyramine, colestipol, which also is a binding resin, can be tried. Long-term treatment with bile acid binders may lead to decompensated bile acid loss, insufficient micelle formation, and steatorrhea. In patients with steatorrhea, the diarrhea may respond to a low-fat diet (about 40 g fat per day).

Many patients with diarrhea-predominant IBD benefit from nonspecific antidiarrheal therapy. Opiate drugs, such as loperamide and diphenoxylate, primarily act by slowing intestinal transit, allowing more contact time for absorption to take place.[126,127] They also increase the tone of the anal sphincter and help anal continence. Especially for patients with postresection diarrhea, antidiarrheal drugs can be of great benefit. Initially, a low dose (eg, 4 mg of loperamide per day) should be given. Then, dosage adjustments can be made by the patient increasing or decreasing the medication according to their needs until the individual optimal level is achieved. In 1 study,[128] this treatment regime resulted in a decrease in daily stool weight from 800 g to 480 g; most of the patients had ileocolonic resection because of CD and the median dose of loperamide ingested was 6 mg per day. Some patients prefer routine dosing, others take antidiarrheals on an as-needed basis, for example before a meal when postprandial diarrhea is a problem, or at nighttime to avoid nocturnal diarrhea, or before travel or social events. If treatment with loperamide or diphenoxylate with atropine fails, more potent opiates, such as codeine and opium, may be tried. Because of the potential of abuse, use of these opiates has to be monitored closely and they must not be prescribed to patients with a history of drug abuse or addiction. Tincture of opium is typically given in a dose of 5 to 20 drops 4 times a day (10 mg morphine/mL); the typical adult dose of codeine is 15 to 60 mg 4 times a day. Opiate drugs have also been effective in the treatment of ileostomy diarrhea[129] and in reducing stool frequency and stool output in colectomized patients with an ileoanal pouch.[130] Tolerance of antimotility drugs can be limited when they induce excessive bloating and abdominal distension. Opiate antidiarrheal drugs should be avoided in patients with fever, abdominal tenderness, or when there is evidence of obstruction or colonic dilatation. They should also be avoided in cases of infection with *Clostridium difficile*, and in patients with bloody diarrhea and suspected invasive bacterial enterocolitis. In patients with acute ulcerative colitis as well as in severely ill patients, opiate drugs can precipitate toxic megacolon.

Bulking agents such as psyllium, methylcellulose, or calcium polycarbophil can also be helpful in alleviating diarrheal symptoms. These agents interact with fecal water and alter the texture and consistency of the stool without reducing stool weight.[131] A moderate increase in consistency (eg, from watery to semiliquid) may be sufficient to improve anal continence in some patients. Patients with distal colitis often have disturbed proximal motility and may benefit from fiber supplementation and antiinflammatory treatment of distal disease.[132] Bulking agents should not be given to patients with high-grade intestinal strictures because they can obstruct the bowel.

REFERENCES

1. Frøslie KF, Jahnsen J, Moum BA, et al. Mucosal healing in inflammatory bowel disease: results from a Norwegian population-based cohort. Gastroenterology 2007;133:412–22.
2. Schiller LR. Microscopic colitis syndrome: lymphocytic colitis and collagenous colitis. Semin Gastrointest Dis 1999;10:145–55.
3. Krejs GJ, Fordtran JS. Physiology and pathophysiology of ion and water movement in the human intestine. In: Sleisinger M, Fordtran JS, editors. Gastrointestinal disease. 2nd edition. Philadelphia, London, Toronto: Saunders; 1978. p. 297–312.
4. Wenzl HH, Fine KD, Schiller LR, et al. Determinants of decreased fecal consistency in patients with diarrhea. Gastroenterology 1995;108:1729–38.
5. Debongnie JC, Phillips SF. Capacity of the human colon to absorb fluid. Gastroenterology 1978;74:698–703.
6. Lindström CG. "Collagenous colitis" with watery diarrhoea: a new entity? Pathol Eur 1976;11:87–9.
7. Read NW, Krejs GJ, Read MG, et al. Chronic diarrhea of unknown origin. Gastroenterology 1980;78:264–71.

8. Lazenby AJ, Yardley JH, Giardiello FM, et al. Lymphocytic (microscopic) colitis: a comparative histopathologic study, with particular reference to collagenous colitis. Hum Pathol 1989;20:18–28.

9. Schiller LR, Sellin JH. Diarrhea. In: Feldman M, Friedman LS, Brandt LJ, editors. Sleisenger and Fordtran's gastrointestinal and liver disease. 9th edition. Philadelphia: WB Saunders; 2010. p. 211–32.

10. Fine KD, Seidel RH, Do K. The prevalence, anatomic distribution, and diagnosis of colonic causes of chronic diarrhea. Gastrointest Endosc 2000;51:318–26.

11. Pardi DS, Loftus EV Jr, Smyrk TC, et al. The epidemiology of microscopic colitis: a population based study in Olmsted County, Minnesota. Gut 2007;56:504–8.

12. Williams JJ, Kaplan GG, Makhija S, et al. Microscopic colitis-defining incidence rates and risk factors: a population-based study. Clin Gastroenterol Hepatol 2008;6:35–40.

13. Olesen M, Eriksson S, Bohr J, et al. Microscopic colitis: a common diarrhoeal disease. An epidemiological study in Orebro, Sweden, 1993-1998. Gut 2004; 53:346–50.

14. Jarnerot G, Tysk C, Bohr J, et al. Collagenous colitis and fecal stream diversion. Gastroenterology 1995;109:449–55.

15. Beaugerie L, Pardi DS. Review article: drug-induced microscopic colitis–proposal for a scoring system and review of the literature. Aliment Pharmacol Ther 2005;22:277–84.

16. Stewart M, Andrews CN, Urbanski S, et al. The association of coeliac disease and microscopic colitis: a large population-based study. Aliment Pharmacol Ther 2011;33:1340–9.

17. Bohr J, Tysk C, Eriksson S, et al. Collagenous colitis: a retrospective study of clinical presentation and treatment in 163 patients. Gut 1996;39:846–51.

18. Olesen M, Eriksson S, Bohr J, et al. Lymphocytic colitis: a retrospective clinical study of 199 Swedish patients. Gut 2004;53:536–41.

19. Pardi DS, Ramnath VR, Loftus EV Jr, et al. Lymphocytic colitis: clinical features, treatment, and outcomes. Am J Gastroenterol 2002;97:2829–33.

20. Fine KD, Do K, Schulte K, et al. High prevalence of celiac sprue-like HLA-DQ genes and enteropathy in patients with the microscopic colitis syndrome. Am J Gastroenterol 2000;95:1974–82.

21. Schiller LR. Pathophysiology and treatment of microscopic-colitis syndrome. Lancet 2000;355:1198–9.

22. Bo-Linn GW, Vendrell DD, Lee E, et al. An evaluation of the significance of microscopic colitis in patients with chronic diarrhea. J Clin Invest 1985;75:1559–69.

23. Rask-Madsen J, Grove O, Hansen MG, et al. Colonic transport of water and electrolytes in a patient with secretory diarrhea due to collagenous colitis. Dig Dis Sci 1983;28:1141–6.

24. Burgel N, Bojarski C, Mankertz J, et al. Mechanisms of diarrhea in collagenous colitis. Gastroenterology 2002;123:433–43.

25. Lee E, Schiller LR, Fordtran JS. Quantification of colonic lamina propria cells by means of a morphometric point-counting method. Gastroenterology 1988;94:409–18.

26. Lee E, Schiller LR, Vendrell D, et al. Subepithelial collagen table thickness in colon specimens from patients with microscopic colitis and collagenous colitis. Gastroenterology 1992;103:1790–6.

27. Wang KK, Perrault J, Carpenter HA, et al. Collagenous colitis. A clinicopathologic correlation. Mayo Clin Proc 1987;62:665–71.

28. Ung KA, Gillberg R, Kilander A, et al. Role of bile acids and bile acid binding agents in patients with collagenous colitis. Gut 2000;46:170–5.

29. Ung KA, Kilander A, Nilsson O, et al. Long-term course in collagenous colitis and the impact of bile acid malabsorption and bile acid sequestrants on histopathology and clinical features. Scand J Gastroenterol 2001;36:601–9.

30. Schiller LR, Bilhartz LE, Santa Ana CA, et al. Comparison of endogenous and radiolabeled bile acid excretion in patients with idiopathic chronic diarrhea. Gastroenterology 1990;98:1036–43.

31. Koskela RM, Niemelä SE, Karttunen TJ, et al. Clinical characteristics of collagenous and lymphocytic colitis. Scand J Gastroenterol 2004;39:837–45.

32. Fine KD, Lee EL. Efficacy of open-label bismuth subsalicylate for the treatment of microscopic colitis. Gastroenterology 1998;114:29–36.

33. Fernandez-Banares F, Salas A, Esteve M, et al. Collagenous and lymphocytic colitis. evaluation of clinical and histological features, response to treatment, and long-term follow-up. Am J Gastroenterol 2003;98:340–7.

34. Chande N, Driman DK, Reynolds RP. Collagenous colitis and lymphocytic colitis: patient characteristics and clinical presentation. Scand J Gastroenterol 2005;40:343–7.

35. Mullhaupt B, Guller U, Anabitarte M, et al. Lymphocytic colitis: clinical presentation in long term course. Gut 1998;43:629–33.

36. Walter SA, Münch A, Ost A, et al. Anorectal function in patients with collagenous colitis in active and clinically quiescent phase, in comparison with healthy controls. Neurogastroenterol Motil 2010;22:534–8.

37. Fine KD, Schiller LR. AGA technical review on the evaluation and management of chronic diarrhea. Gastroenterology 1999;116:1464–86.

38. Offner FA, Jao RV, Lewin KJ, et al. Collagenous colitis: a study of the distribution of morphological abnormalities and their histological detection. Hum Pathol 1999;30:451–7.

39. ASGE Standards of Practice Committee, Shen B, Khan K, Ikenberry SO, et al. The role of endoscopy in the management of patients with diarrhea. Gastrointest Endosc 2010;71:887–92.

40. Yantiss RK, Odze RD. Optimal approach to obtaining mucosal biopsies for assessment of inflammatory disorders of the gastrointestinal tract. Am J Gastroenterol 2009;104:774–83.

41. Chande N, MacDonald JK, McDonald JW. Interventions for treating microscopic colitis: a Cochrane Inflammatory Bowel Disease and Functional Bowel Disorders Review Group systematic review of randomized trials. Am J Gastroenterol 2009; 104:235–41.

42. Fine KD, Ogunji F, Lee EL, et al. Randomized, double-blind, placebo-controlled trial of bismuth subsalicylate for microscopic colitis [abstract]. Gastroenterology 1999;116:A880.

43. Fernandez-Bañares F, Esteve M, Salas A, et al. Bile acid malabsorption in microscopic colitis and in previously unexplained functional chronic diarrhea. Dig Dis Sci 2001;46:2231–8.

44. Calabrese C, Fabbri A, Areni A, et al. Mesalazine with or without cholestyramine in the treatment of microscopic colitis: randomized controlled trial. J Gastroenterol Hepatol 2007;22:809–14.

45. Miehlke S, Madisch A, Kupcinskas L, et al. Double-blind, double-dummy, placebo-controlled, multicenter trial of budesonide and measlamine in collagenous colitis [abstract]. Gastroenterology 2012;142(S1):211.

46. Munck LK, Kjeldsen J, Philipsen E, et al. Incomplete remission with short-term prednisolone treatment in collagenous colitis: a randomized study. Scand J Gastroenterol 2003;38:606–10.

47. Pardi DS, Loftus EV Jr, Tremaine WJ, et al. Treatment of refractory microscopic colitis with azathioprine and 6-mercaptopurine. Gastroenterology 2001;120: 1483–4.

48. Riddell J, Hillman L, Chiragakis L, et al. Collagenous colitis: oral low-dose methotrexate for patients with difficult symptoms: long-term outcomes. J Gastroenterol Hepatol 2007;22:1589–93.

49. Esteve M, Mahadevan U, Sainz E, et al. Efficacy of anti-TNF therapies in refractory severe microscopic colitis. J Crohns Colitis 2011;5:612–8.

50. Münch A, Ignatova S, Ström M. Adalimumab in budesonide and methotrexate refractory collagenous colitis. Scand J Gastroenterol 2012;47:59–63.

51. Riaz AA, Pitt J, Stirling RW, et al. Restorative proctocolectomy for collagenous colitis. J R Soc Med 2000;93:261.

52. Yardley JH, Lazenby AJ, Giardiello FM, et al. Collagenous, "microscopic," lymphocytic, and other gentler and more subtle forms of colitis. Hum Pathol 1990;21:1089–91.

53. Rao SSC, Holdsworth CD, Read NW. Symptoms and stool patterns in patients with ulcerative colitis. Gut 1988;29:342–5.

54. Harris J, Shields R. Absorption and secretion of water and electrolytes by the intact human colon in diffuse untreated proctocolitis. Gut 1970;11:27–33.

55. Rask-Madsen J, Hammersgaard EA, Knudsen E. Rectal electrolyte transport and mucosal permeability in ulcerative colitis and Crohn's disease. J Lab Clin Med 1973;81:342–53.

56. Allgayer H, Kruis W, Paumgartner G, et al. Inverse relationship between colonic (Na+ + K+)-ATPase activity and degree of mucosal inflammation in inflammatory bowel disease. Dig Dis Sci 1988;33:417–22.

57. Sandle GI, Higgs N, Crowe P, et al. Cellular basis for defective electrolyte transport in inflamed human colon. Gastroenterology 1990;99:97–105.

58. Greig ER, Boot-Handford RP, Mani V, et al. Decreased expression of apical Na+ channels and basolateral Na+, K+-ATPase in ulcerative colitis. J Pathol 2004; 204:84–92.

59. Hawker PC, McKay JS, Turnberg LA. Electrolyte transport across colonic mucosa from patients with inflammatory bowel disease. Gastroenterology 1980;79:508–11.

60. Amasheh S, Barmeyer C, Koch CS, et al. Cytokine-dependent transcriptional down-regulation of epithelial sodium channel in ulcerative colitis. Gastroenterology 2004;126:1711–20.

61. Sullivan S, Alex P, Dassopoulos T, et al. Downregulation of sodium transporters and NHERF proteins in IBD patients and mouse colitis models: potential contributors to IBD-associated diarrhea. Inflamm Bowel Dis 2009;15:261–74.

62. Gitter AH, Wullstein F, Fromm M, et al. Epithelial barrier defects in ulcerative colitis: characterization and quantification by electrophysiological imaging. Gastroenterology 2001;121:1320–8.

63. Schmitz H, Barmeyer C, Fromm M, et al. Altered tight junction structure contributes to the impaired epithelial barrier function in ulcerative colitis. Gastroenterology 1999;116:301–9.

64. Krejs GJ, Fordtran JS, Fahrenkrug J, et al. Effect of VIP infusion in water and ion transport in the human jejunum. Gastroenterology 1980;78:722–7.

65. Sandle GI. Pathogenesis of diarrhea in ulcerative colitis: new views on an old problem. J Clin Gastroenterol 2005;39(Suppl 2):S49–52.

66. Gooptu D, Truelove SC, Warner GT. Absorption of electrolytes from the colon in cases of ulcerative colitis and in control subjects. Gut 1969;10:555–61.

67. Head LH, Heaton JW Jr, Kivel RM. Absorption of water and electrolytes in Crohn's disease of the colon. Gastroenterology 1969;56:571–9.
68. Allan R, Steinberg DM, Dixon K, et al. Changes in the bidirectional sodium flux across the intestinal mucosa in Crohn's disease. Gut 1975;16:201–4.
69. Atwell JD, Duthie HL. The absorption of water, sodium, and potassium from the ileum of humans showing the effects of regional enteritis. Gastroenterology 1964;46:16–22.
70. Archampong EQ, Harris J, Clark CG. The absorption and secretion of water and electrolytes across the healthy and the diseased human colonic mucosa measured in vitro. Gut 1972;11:880–6.
71. Carethers JM, McDonnell WM, Owyang C, et al. Massive secretory diarrhea and pseudo-obstruction as the initial presentation of Crohn's disease. J Clin Gastroenterol 1996;23:55–9.
72. Zeissig S, Bergann T, Fromm A. Altered ENaC expression leads to impaired sodium absorption in the noninflamed intestine in Crohn's disease. Gastroenterology 2008;134:1436–47.
73. Musch MW, Clarke LL, Mamah D, et al. T cell activation causes diarrhea by increasing intestinal permeability and inhibiting epithelial Na+/K+-ATPase. J Clin Invest 2002;110:1739–47.
74. Clayburgh DR, Musch MW, Leitges M, et al. Coordinated epithelial NHE3 inhibition and barrier dysfunction are required for TNF-mediated diarrhea in vivo. J Clin Invest 2006;116:2682–94.
75. Montgomery RD, Frazer AC, Hood C, et al. Studies of intestinal fermentation in ulcerative colitis. Gut 1968;9:521–6.
76. Rao SS, Read NW, Holdsworth CD. Is the diarrhoea in ulcerative colitis related to impaired colonic salvage of carbohydrate? Gut 1987;28:1090–4.
77. Reddy SN, Bazzocchi G, Chan S, et al. Colonic motility and transit in health and ulcerative colitis. Gastroenterology 1991;101:1289–97.
78. Rao SS, Read NW, Brown C, et al. Studies on the mechanism of bowel disturbance in ulcerative colitis. Gastroenterology 1987;93:934–40.
79. Rao SS, Read NW. Gastrointestinal motility in patients with ulcerative colitis. Scand J Gastroenterol Suppl 1990;172:22–8.
80. Hofmann AF. The continuing importance of bile acids in liver and intestinal disease. Arch Intern Med 1999;159(22):2647–58.
81. Hofmann AF, Poley JR. Role of bile acid malabsorption in pathogenesis of diarrhea and steatorrhea in patients with ileal resection. I. Response to cholestyramine or replacement of dietary long chain triglyceride by medium chain triglyceride. Gastroenterology 1972;62:918–34.
82. Jacobsen O, Højgaard L, Hylander Møller E, et al. Effect of enterocoated cholestyramine on bowel habit after ileal resection: a double blind crossover study. Br Med J (Clin Res Ed) 1985;290:1315–8.
83. Poley JR, Hofmann AF. Role of fat maldigestion in pathogenesis of steatorrhea in ileal resection. Fat digestion after two sequential test meals with and without cholestyramine. Gastroenterology 1976;71:38–44.
84. Schiller LR. Diarrhea following small bowel resection. In: Bayless TM, Hanauer SB, editors. Advanced therapy of inflammatory bowel diseases. Hamilton (Ontario): BC Decker; 2001. p. 471–4.
85. Andersson H, Isaksson B, Sjögren B. Fat-reduced diet in the symptomatic treatment of small bowel disease: metabolic studies in patients with Crohn's disease and in other patients subjected to ileal resection. Gut 1974;15:351–9.

86. Fordtran JS, Bunch F, Davis GR. Ox bile treatment of severe steatorrhea in an ileectomy-ileostomy patient. Gastroenterology 1982;82:564–8.
87. Little KH, Schiller LR, Bilhartz LE, et al. Treatment of severe steatorrhea with ox bile in an ileectomy patient with residual colon. Dig Dis Sci 1992;37:929–33.
88. Gruy-Kapral C, Little KH, Fordtran JS, et al. Conjugated bile acid replacement therapy for short-bowel syndrome. Gastroenterology 1999;116:15–21.
89. Hammer HF, Fine KD, Santa Ana CA, et al. Carbohydrate malabsorption. Its measurement and its contribution to diarrhea. J Clin Invest 1990;86:1936–44.
90. Hammer HF, Santa Ana CA, Schiller LR, et al. Studies of osmotic diarrhea induced in normal subjects by ingestion of polyethylene glycol and lactulose. J Clin Invest 1989;84:1056–62.
91. Caspary WF. Diarrhoea associated with carbohydrate malabsorption. Clin Gastroenterol 1986;15:631–55.
92. Schiller LR. Chronic diarrhea of obscure origin. In: Field M, editor. Diarrheal diseases. New York: Elsevier; 1991. p. 219–38.
93. Pironi L, Callegari C, Cornia GL, et al. Lactose malabsorption in adult patients with Crohn's disease. Am J Gastroenterol 1988;83:1267–71.
94. Barrett JS, Irving PM, Shepherd SJ, et al. Comparison of the prevalence of fructose and lactose malabsorption across chronic intestinal disorders. Aliment Pharmacol Ther 2009;30:165–74.
95. Mishkin B, Yalovsky M, Mishkin S. Increased prevalence of lactose malabsorption in Crohn's disease patients at low risk for lactose malabsorption based on ethnic origin. Am J Gastroenterol 1997;92:1148–53.
96. von Tirpitz C, Kohn C, Steinkamp M, et al. Lactose intolerance in active Crohn's disease: clinical value of duodenal lactase analysis. J Clin Gastroenterol 2002;34:49–53.
97. Eherer AJ, Fordtran JS. Fecal osmotic gap and pH in experimental diarrhea of various causes. Gastroenterology 1992;103:545–51.
98. Broe PJ, Cameron JL. Surgical management of ileosigmoid fistulas in Crohn's disease. Am J Surg 1982;143:611–3.
99. Levy C, Tremaine WJ. Management of internal fistulas in Crohn's disease. Inflamm Bowel Dis 2002;8:106–11.
100. Klaus J, Spaniol U, Adler G, et al. Small intestinal bacterial overgrowth mimicking acute flare as a pitfall in patients with Crohn's disease. BMC Gastroenterol 2009;9:61.
101. Beeken WL, Kanich RE. Microbial flora of the upper small bowel in Crohn's disease. Gastroenterology 1973;65:390–7.
102. Mishkin D, Boston FM, Blank D, et al. The glucose breath test, a diagnostic test for small bowel stricture (s) in Crohn's disease. Dig Dis Sci 2002;47:489–94.
103. Castiglione F, Del Vecchio Blanco G, Rispo A, et al. Orocecal transit time and bacterial overgrowth in patients with Crohn's disease. J Clin Gastroenterol 2000;31:63–6.
104. Mylonaki M, Langmead L, Pantes A, et al. Enteric infection in relapse of inflammatory bowel disease: importance of microbiological examination of stool. Eur J Gastroenterol Hepatol 2004;16:775–8.
105. Issa M, Vijayapal A, Graham MB, et al. Impact of *Clostridium difficile* on inflammatory bowel disease. Clin Gastroenterol Hepatol 2007;5:345–51.
106. Rodemann JF, Dubberke ER, Reske KA, et al. Incidence of *Clostridium difficile* infection in inflammatory bowel disease. Clin Gastroenterol Hepatol 2007;5:339–44.
107. Ananthakrishnan AN, McGinley EL, Binion DG. Excess hospitalisation burden associated with *Clostridium difficile* in patients with inflammatory bowel disease. Gut 2008;57:205–10.

108. Kornbluth A, Sachar DB, Practice Parameters Committee of the American College of Gastroenterology. Ulcerative colitis practice guidelines in adults: American College Of Gastroenterology, Practice Parameters Committee. Am J Gastroenterol 2010;105:501–23.
109. Lichtenstein GR, Hanauer SB, Sandborn WJ. Practice Parameters Committee of American College of Gastroenterology. Management of Crohn's disease in adults. Am J Gastroenterol 2009;104:465–83.
110. Epple HJ. Therapy- and non-therapy-dependent infectious complications in inflammatory bowel disease. Dig Dis 2009;27:555–9.
111. Goldstein F, DiMarino AJ Jr. Diarrhea as a side effect of mesalamine treatment for inflammatory bowel disease. J Clin Gastroenterol 2000;31:60–2.
112. Fine KD, Sarles HE Jr, Cryer B. Diarrhea associated with mesalamine in a patient with chronic nongranulomatous enterocolitis. N Engl J Med 1998;338:923–5.
113. Marbet U, Schmid I. Severe life-threatening diarrhea caused by azathioprine but not by 6-mercaptopurine. Digestion 2001;63:139–42.
114. Cox J, Daneshmend TK, Hawkey CJ, et al. Devastating diarrhoea caused by azathioprine: management difficulty in inflammatory bowel disease. Gut 1988; 29:686–8.
115. Bayless TM, Harris ML. Inflammatory bowel disease and irritable bowel syndrome. Med Clin North Am 1990;74:21–8.
116. Stange EF, Travis SP, Vermeire S, et al. European evidence-based Consensus on the diagnosis and management of ulcerative colitis: definitions and diagnosis. J Crohns Colitis 2008;2:1–23.
117. Fine KD, Fordtran JS. The effect of diarrhea on fecal fat excretion. Gastroenterology 1992;102:1936–9.
118. Nyhlin H, Merrick MV, Eastwood MA. Bile acid malabsorption in Crohn's disease and indications for its assessment using SeHCAT. Gut 1994;35:90–3.
119. Modigliani R, Mary JY, Simon JF, et al. Clinical, biological, and endoscopic picture of attacks of Crohn's disease. Evolution on prednisolone. Groupe d'Etude Thérapeutique des Affections Inflammatoires Digestives. Gastroenterology 1990;98:811–8.
120. Van Assche G, Dignass A, Panes J, et al. The second European evidence-based Consensus on the diagnosis and management of Crohn's disease: definitions and diagnosis. J Crohns Colitis 2010;4:7–27.
121. Travis SP, Stange EF, Lémann M, et al. European evidence-based Consensus on the management of ulcerative colitis: current management. J Crohns Colitis 2008;2:24–62.
122. Dignass A, Van Assche G, Lindsay JO, et al. The second European evidence-based Consensus on the diagnosis and management of Crohn's disease: current management. J Crohns Colitis 2010;4:28–62.
123. Rahier JF, Ben-Horin S, Chowers Y, et al. European evidence-based Consensus on the prevention, diagnosis and management of opportunistic infections in inflammatory bowel disease. J Crohns Colitis 2009;3:47–91.
124. Castiglione F, Rispso A, Di Girolamo E, et al. Antibiotic treatment of small bowel bacterial overgrowth in patients with Crohn's disease. Aliment Pharmacol Ther 2003;18:1107–11.
125. Biancone L, Vernia P, Agostini D, et al. Effect of rifaximin on intestinal bacterial overgrowth in Crohn's disease as assessed by the H2-Glucose Breath Test. Curr Med Res Opin 2000;16:14–20.
126. Schiller LR, Davis GR, Santa Ana CA, et al. Studies of the mechanism of the antidiarrheal effect of codeine. J Clin Invest 1982 Nov;70:999–1008.

127. Schiller LR, Santa Ana CA, Morawski SG, et al. Mechanism of the antidiarrheal effect of loperamide. Gastroenterology 1984;86:1475–80.
128. Mainguet P, Fiasse R. Double-blind placebo-controlled study of loperamide (Imodium) in chronic diarrhoea caused by ileocolic disease or resection. Gut 1977;18:575–9.
129. DuPont AW, Sellin JH. Ileostomy diarrhea. Curr Treat Options Gastroenterol 2006;9:39–48.
130. Herbst F, Kamm MA, Nicholls RJ. Effects of loperamide on ileoanal pouch function. Br J Surg 1998;85:1428–32.
131. Eherer AJ, Santa Ana CA, Porter J, et al. Effect of psyllium, calcium polycarbophil, and wheat bran on secretory diarrhea induced by phenolphthalein. Gastroenterology 1993;104:1007–12.
132. Griffin MG, Miner PB. Review article: refractory distal colitis–explanation and options. Aliment Pharmacol Ther 1996;10:39–48.

Diarrhea in the Immunocompromised Patient

Elisabeth Krones, MD, Christoph Högenauer, MD*

KEYWORDS

- HIV • GVHD • *Clostridium difficile* • CMV • Cryptosporidiosis • HSCT • Diarrhea
- Colitis

KEY POINTS

- Diagnostic management of diarrhea in immunocompromised conditions includes clinical assessment, drug history, microbiological stool examination, and endoscopy.
- *Clostridium difficile* is the most common bacterial pathogen causing diarrhea in patients infected with human immunodeficiency virus and in other immunocompromised patients.
- Idiopathic AIDS enteropathy improves with highly active antiretroviral therapy and increasing CD4 counts.
- Cytomegalovirus disease is a major cause of morbidity and mortality in immunocompromised patients and may be confirmed by endoscopic biopsy and histologic analysis, including immunologic staining.
- Intestinal graft-versus-host disease is primarily treated with glucocorticoids.

INTRODUCTION

Diarrhea is a common problem in patients with immunocompromising conditions. The etiologic spectrum (**Tables 1** and **2**) differs significantly from patients with diarrhea who have a normal immune system. Especially opportunistic pathogens are frequent causative agents. Furthermore, some conditions, such as intestinal graft-versus-host disease (GVHD) or neutropenic enterocolitis, occur only in these patients. For correct diagnosis and therapy, it is therefore important to be familiar with the various conditions that need to be considered in diarrhea in an immunocompromised patient. This article reviews the most important causes of diarrhea in these patients, ranging from infectious causes to noninfectious causes of diarrhea in the setting of HIV infection as a model for other conditions of immunosuppression. It also deals with diarrhea in specific situations, eg, after hematopoietic stem cell or solid organ transplantation,

The authors have no conflicts to disclose.

Division of Gastroenterology and Hepatology, Department of Internal Medicine, Medical University of Graz, Auenbruggerplatz 15, A-8036 Graz, Austria

* Corresponding author.

E-mail address: christoph.hoegenauer@medunigraz.at

http://dx.doi.org/10.1016/j.gtc.2012.06.009
0889-8553/12/$ – see front matter © 2012 Elsevier Inc. All rights reserved.

gastro.theclinics.com

Table 1	
Infectious agents causing diarrhea in immunocompromised patients	
Bacteria	*Salmonella* spp
	Shigella spp
	Campylobacter spp
	Clostridium difficile
	Chlamydia trachomatis
	Pathogenic *Escherichia coli*
Mycobacteria	*Mycobacterium avium* complex
	Mycobacterium tuberculosis
Parasites	*Cryptosporidium* spp
	Cytoisospora belli
	Giardia lamblia
	Entamoeba histolytica
	Blastocystis hominis
	Cyclospora spp
	Strongyloides stercoralis
Viruses	*Cytomegalovirus*
	Adenovirus spp
	Rotavirus spp
	Norovirus
	Herpes simplex
	Human immunodeficiency virus
Fungi	*Microsporidium*
	Histoplasmosis
	Candida spp
Other	Neutropenic enterocolitis

Table 2	
Noninfectious causes of diarrhea in immunocompromised patients	
Human immunodeficiency virus–associated diarrhea	Idiopathic AIDS enteropathy
	Neoplasms (Lymphoma, Kaposi sarcoma)
	Highly active antiretroviral therapy
	Pancreatic insufficiency
Drug-induced diarrhea	Antibiotics
	Azathioprine
	Chemotherapeutics
	Cyclosporine A
	Methotrexate
	Mycophenolate mofetil
	Sirolimus
	Tacrolimus
Graft versus host disease	After allogeneic stem cell transplantation
	After autologous stem cell transplantation
	After solid organ transplantation
	After blood transfusions
Other	Cord colitis syndrome
	Inflammatory bowel disease
	Gluten-sensitive enteropathy
	Idiopathic forms of enteritis and colitis
	Posttransplantation lymphoproliferative diseases

diarrhea induced by immunosuppressive drugs, and diarrhea in congenital immuno-deficiency syndromes.

DIARRHEA AS A CONSEQUENCE OF INFECTION WITH HUMAN IMMUNODEFICIENCY VIRUS

The gastrointestinal tract plays an important role in human immunodeficiency virus (HIV) infection because almost all HIV-infected hosts develop gastrointestinal compli-cations during the course of their disease.[1] In Africa, HIV infection was formerly called "slim disease" because of watery diarrhea, weight loss, malnutrition, and a wasting away followed by death.[2,3] Before the era of highly active antiretroviral therapy (HAART), diarrhea, which increases in frequency and severity as immune function deteriorates,[4] complicated the clinical course of 40% to 80% of HIV-infected patients.[5–7] Substantial diarrhea has been reported to occur in about half of the HIV-infected individuals in the United States; however, the prevalence of HIV-associated diarrhea is much higher in developing countries.[3] Besides noninfectious causes, like idiopathic AIDS enteropathy or drug-induced diarrhea in the era of HAART, diarrhea in HIV-infected patients is most frequently caused by opportunistic infections owing to alterations in the mucosal immune system.[5,8] Apart from infectious pathogens, diarrhea in patients with AIDS can be caused by neoplasms (eg, lymphoma, Kaposi sarcoma) or pancreatic disease.[8] However, there is lack of controlled prospective studies regarding the etiology of HIV-associated diarrhea in countries with the highest prevalence of HIV.[5] Diagnostic management of HIV-associated diarrhea includes clinical assessment of the underlying disease (eg, CD4 count, HIV viral load), drug history, microbiological stool examination (eg, microscopy for ova, cysts and parasites, bacterial culture, virology and protozoan polymerase chain reaction [PCR]) as well as endoscopic examination including biopsies (eg, histology, cytomegalovirus [CMV] PCR, malignancies).[5] Exact endoscopic evaluation, including colonoscopy with intubation and biopsy of the terminal ileum together with endoscopy of the upper gastrointestinal tract, allows the identification of specific path-ogens in approximately 50% of the patients formerly classified to have stool-study–negative idiopathic diarrhea[3,9]; however, a full endoscopic workup is not necessary in every patient but should be especially considered in patients with a functionally disabling diarrhea of unclear etiology.[3] Clinical presentation of HIV-associated diar-rhea may vary depending on the area of the gastrointestinal tract involved. Diarrhea from small bowel affection usually results in voluminous postprandial diarrhea and weight loss, whereas diarrhea from large bowel disease ("colitic diarrhea") is charac-terized by frequent small-volume stools with or without visible blood or mucous.[3]

INFECTIOUS DIARRHEA IN IMMUNOCOMPROMISED PATIENTS

Patients with immunocompromised states (eg, HIV infection, solid organ transplanta-tion, stem cell transplantation, hematologic malignancies) are at a high risk for severe gastrointestinal infections caused by viruses, bacteria and parasites. Compared with healthy hosts, these infectious diseases frequently run a more severe clinical course in immunocompromised patients and are associated with significant morbidity and mortality throughout the world.[10–12] Moreover, severe diseases in immunosuppressed hosts may be caused by pathogens that rarely cause symptomatic infection in healthy individuals.[12] Infectious diarrhea in HIV-infected patients may be caused by a broad spectrum of organisms. Impaired function of the mucosal immune system may predis-pose to a more severe clinical course of enteric infections with common pathogens, such as *Salmonella* spp, *Shigella* spp, or *Campylobacter*. The most common infectious agents of HIV-associated diarrhea include bacteria such as *Salmonella* spp, *Clostridium difficile, Mycobacterium tuberculosis,* and nontuberculous mycobacteria; viruses such as *Cytomegalovirus;* and fungal and parasitic infections. More detailed information on the different pathogens is provided in the following sections.

PARASITIC INFECTIONS

Parasites causing diarrhea in HIV and other immunocompromising conditions include parasites previously described to have pathogenic potential in healthy hosts (ie, *Giardia lamblia, Entamoeba histolytica, Blastocystis hominis,* and *Strongyloides stercoralis*), as well as parasites usually not causing disease in healthy humans (ie, *Cryptosporidium* spp, *Isospora belli, Cyclospora cayetanensis*).[5]

Cryptosporidiosis

Cryptosporidium spp are tiny intracellular protozoan parasites that infect the gastrointestinal epithelium of vertebrates.[13] Most human infections are caused by *Cryptosporidium hominis* and *Cryptosporidium parvum*[14] and mainly affect immunocompromised individuals or immunocompetent children younger than 5.[15,16] *Cryptosporidium* is widespread in the developing world.[17] Oral ingestion of an infectious dose of oocysts results in the formation of sporozoites in the intestinal lumen. Sporozoites subsequently attach to the intestinal epithelium, triggering elongation and fusion of epithelial cell microvilli enclosing the sporozoite within a vacuole.[18] Sporozoites then develop into merozoites, which replicate and invade neighboring cells.[13] *Cryptosporidium* spp infection usually involves the small bowel. Enteric illness ranges from self-limiting diarrhea in immunocompetent hosts to severe prolonged enteritis refractory to treatment in immunocompromised individuals. The latter is the most common clinical feature of cryptosporidial infection in humans.[19] *Cryptosporidium* spp infection may additionally involve the respiratory epithelium or the biliary tract.[8] Clinical manifestations of cryptosporidiosis depend on the immune-status of the infected host. *Cryptosporidium* spp has especially been associated with chronic diarrhea, decreased quality of life, and shortened survival in HIV-infected patients.[20–24] Morbidity from cryptosporidiosis has markedly decreased in the era of HAART but is still a problem in developing countries with limited access to this therapy.[22–27]

Diagnosis is established by stool testing using specific stains, PCR or small bowel or rectal biopsies. Oocyts may be detected with a modified acid-fast stain of the stool, enzyme-linked immunosorbent assay (ELISA) or direct fluorescence antibody tests. Although there is some evidence for effectiveness of nitazoxanide, administered 500 mg twice daily until clinical symptoms resolve and oocysts are eliminated from the stool,[28] there are currently no further data supporting the effectiveness of chemotherapeutic agents in the treatment of cryptosporidiosis in immunocompromised patients.[15] Treatment should primarily comprise supportive management, including rehydration, electrolyte replacement, and antimotility agents.[15] In HIV-infected patients, HAART is the most important treatment to improve the immune function and the CD4 counts.[13]

Strongyloidiasis

Strongyloidiasis is a parasitic infection caused by the intestinal nematode *Strongyloides*. The most frequently found species pathogenic for humans, resulting in abdominal pain and diarrhea worldwide, is *Strongyloides stercoralis*,[29] which is endemic to tropical and subtropical regions.[30] After penetrating the skin and entering circulation, the filariform larvae proceed to the lungs, penetrate the alveoli, ascend the tracheobronchial tree and are subsequently swallowed. In the duodenum and jejunum, the larvae mature into adult females that produce up to 40 eggs per day, subsequently releasing the larvae into the intestinal wall.[29,31–34] After migrating into the intestinal lumen, the larvae are passed into feces or mature into filariform larvae that infect the intestinal mucosa or perianal region.[33] In immunocompromised patients (eg, immune deficiency, hematologic malignancies, administration of corticosteroids, HIV infection, diabetes, transplantation, advanced age), a hyperinfection syndrome, which is characterized by detection of increased number of larvae in stool, sputum, and tissue, may increase mortality.[29,32,35,36] Half of the patients with *Strongyloides* infection are asymptomatic.[29,32] However, the most common clinical manifestations are related to the gastrointestinal tract and mainly include unspecific symptoms, such as abdominal pain, diarrhea, vomiting, flatulence, and constipation. In advanced cases, paralytic ileus, small bowel obstruction, gastrointestinal bleeding, and protein-losing enteropathy may occur.[29,32,34] In the larvae's migration phase, respiratory symptoms ranging from coughing or wheezing to severe symptoms, such as dyspnea, pleuritic pain, or hemoptysis in case of hyperinfection syndrome, may be seen.[29,32,34] Diagnostic tools include stool testing for ova and parasites, complete blood count to check for eosinophilia, ELISA for *S stercoralis* serology if available, sputum cultures in patients with pulmonary manifestations and suspected hyperinfection syndrome, and small bowel biopsy.[32] The examination of duodenal biopsy specimens for ova and larvae is the most sensitive diagnostic procedure for *S stercoralis*.[31] *S stercoralis* hyperinfection is a cause of severe illness in immunocompromised patients and should be especially considered in patients from areas where this infection is endemic.[31] Treatment options for uncomplicated disease include ivermectin, thiabendazole, and albendazole alone or in combination. Ivermectin, a macrolide like agent that has become the drug of choice in strongyloidiasis, should be given at a dose of 200 µg/kg orally once a day for 1 to 2 days in patients with uncomplicated disease weighing more than 15 kg. If necessary, treatment may be repeated 2 to 3 weeks after the first course.[32] In hyperinfection syndrome and disseminated disease, ivermectin is recommended to be administered daily until symptoms resolve and stool tests have been negative for at least 2 weeks.[32] Thiabendazole at a dosage of 25 mg/kg orally twice a day for 3 days may be given as an alternative in complicated infection but has significant adverse events, such as dizziness, nausea, and abdominal pain.[32] Albendazole, a broad-spectrum anthelmintic agent, at a dosage of 10 mg/kg/d for 7 days can be used as an alternative if the previous drugs are not available.[32,37] However, there are limited data on treatment options for hyperinfection or disseminated disease with anthelmintic drugs.[32]

Cytoisosporiasis (Formerly Known as Isosporiasis)

Infection with the protozoan *Cytoisospora belli* (formerly known as *Isospora belli*) commonly runs a benign, asymptomatic, and self-limiting course in immunocompetent patients, whereas in immunocompromised hosts, symptoms may range from watery diarrhea, vomiting, abdominal pain, and weight loss to dehydration often requiring subsequent hospitalization.[26] *Cytoisospora belli* is the only *Cytoisospora* protozoan infecting humans and commonly occurs in tropical and subtropical regions.[38] Most of the cases have been reported in patients with AIDS and kidney or liver transplantation.[26,39–42] Treatment options for Cytoisosporiasis include trimethoprim/sulfamethoxazole (160 mg/800 mg) given orally 4 times a day for 10 days[43] as well as ciprofloxacin (500 mg) twice daily for 7 days as an alternative in case of allergy to sulphonamides.[44]

BACTERIAL INFECTIONS

Although HIV-infected patients are not at an increased risk of developing acute diarrhea from bacterial agents compared with healthy individuals, diarrhea caused by common pathogens, such as *Salmonella* and *Campylobacter jejuni,* runs a more virulent and invasive clinical course in HIV-infected patients.[5,8] Besides *Salmonella* and *Campylobacter* spp leading to prolonged infection and invasive disease, other organisms such as pathogenic *Escherichia coli*, *Shigella* spp, and *Clostridium difficile* have been described as common causative pathogens of infectious diarrhea among HIV-infected individuals.[5] *C difficile* has even been reported to be the most common recognized cause of bacterial diarrhea among HIV-infected individuals.[45]

Campylobacter spp

Bloodstream infection caused by *Campylobacter* is a rare condition and mainly occurs in patients with immune deficiency, hypogammaglobulinemia, HIV infection, malignancy, and solid organ transplantation.[46,47] Before the era of HAART, advanced stage HIV disease was the most important underlying condition in *Campylobacter* bacteremia.[46] Interestingly, *Campylobacter* bacteremia has been reported to have an extra-intestinal origin in approximately 30% of the cases; however, the most common source of bacteremia is found intra-abdominal.[46] Clinical characteristics include fever as the most common clinical symptom, followed by abdominal pain and diarrhea, as well as less frequent complaints such as respiratory symptoms and soft tissue damage.[46]

Salmonella spp

Bloodstream infection with nontyphoid *Salmonella* infection has been reported in heart-transplant recipients.[48] Cases of infection with nontyphoid *Salmonella*, foodborne pathogens causing gastroenteritis, bacteremia, and focal metastatic infection,[49] have also been reported in patients after renal transplantation.[50–55] Clinical presentation of nontyphoid *Salmonella* infection in solid-organ transplant recipients, including febrile enteritis and bloodstream infection, differs from that seen in immunocompetent hosts, where *Salmonella* usually causes nonfebrile gastrointestinal infection.[48]

Chlamydia Trachomatis

Ulcerative rectocolitis mimicking the clinical picture of Crohn's disease in HIV-infected patients may rarely also be caused by gut mucosal infection owing to lymphogranuloma venerum caused by serovars L1 to L3 of *Chlamydia trachomatis,* which is currently reemerging as a sexually transmitted disease.[5,56,57] Diagnosis of bacterial diarrhea may easily be established by stool cultures and blood cultures owing to the high rate of bacteremia in these patients.[8] Antimicrobial treatment should be administered according to identification of specific organisms by culture, as well as local resistance rates.

Mycobacterium spp

Mycobacterial infections with *Mycobacterium tuberculosis* and nontuberculous mycobacteria (eg, *Mycobacterium avium*) may cause gastrointestinal infections presenting with diarrhea in HIV-associated immunosuppression.[58,59] In contrast to infections with *M tuberculosis*, which rarely present with diarrhea, diarrhea it is a common feature in infections with members of the *M avium* complex.[5,60] Disseminated *M avium* complex disease is the most common opportunistic bacterial infection in advanced stage AIDS.[61–65] Although the rate of *M avium* complex infection has declined in the era of HAART, patients with low CD4 counts remain at an increased risk.[66,67] Clinical presentation of *M avium* complex disease includes fever, weight loss, night sweats, fatigue, and watery diarrhea, usually without fecal white blood cells,[2] malabsorption, lymphadenopathy, organomegaly, anemia, and elevated liver enzymes; however, all of these symptoms may also occur during the course of HIV infection either as a symptom of advanced stage HIV infection or with other opportunistic infections.[5,68] Abdominal symptoms, such as pain and diarrhea, have been reported in one-fourth to one-third of patients with *M avium* complex disease.[68] Gastrointestinal infection usually affects the upper gastrointestinal tract (eg, duodenum), which may be suggested at endoscopy by the presence of multiple raised mucosal nodules or yellowish patches (**Fig. 1**A).[69] Less common endoscopic findings include ulceration, edema, erythema, aphthous lesions, or strictures.[70] Diagnosis can be established by endoscopic biopsy. Small-bowel biopsies may show macrophages filled with acid-fast bacilli, similar to Whipple disease.[2] *M avium* infection may also be revealed by blood and stool cultures, although stool cultures have not been suggested to be useful when blood cultures are negative.[68] Preferred treatment regimens for disseminated *M avium* infection are (1) clarithromycin (500 mg twice daily) plus ethambutol (15 mg/kg once daily) with or without rifabutin (300 mg once daily), which has been shown to reduce mortality when added, or (2) azithromycin (500–600 mg once daily) plus ethambutol (15 mg/kg daily).[66] Fluorochinolones (eg, moxifloxacin 400 mg once daily or levofloxacin 500–750 mg once daily) plus ethambutol plus rifabutin have been suggested for patients with clarithromycin-resistant *M avium* infection.[66] Patients with CD4 counts less than 50 cells/mm³ are at increased risk for *M avium* infection, and should receive chemoprophylaxis with azithromycin (1200 mg once per week) or clarithromycin (500 mg twice daily).[66] Alternatively, rifabutin at a dosage of 300 mg once daily or azithromycin at dosages ranging from 500 to 600 mg once daily may be given. Prophylaxis can be stopped when CD4 counts increase to more than 100 cells/mm³.[66]

Clostridium difficile

Clostridium difficile is a gram-positive spore-forming bacterium. Strains producing toxin A and/or toxin B can cause colitis and diarrhea *C difficile* is a common nosocomial infection when hospital inpatients get infected with spores, which often contaminate the hospital environment and hands or instruments of health care workers. The spores of *C difficile* are resistant to alcohol-based disinfectants and can survive in the environment for up to 6 months. Risk factors for *C difficile* infection (CDI) are a previous antibiotic therapy altering the normal intestinal microbiota and its colonization resistance to pathogens, acid-suppressing drugs, especially proton pump inhibitors, advanced age, severe underlying diseases, surgery, and a previous chemotherapy.[71] Immunocompromised

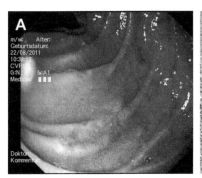 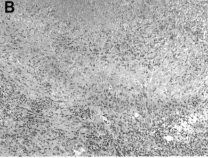

Fig. 1. Endoscopy of the duodenum of a patient with *Mycobacterium avium* infection with the presence of raised mucosal nodules and yellowish patches (*panel A*). Histology of mesenteric lymph nodes showing granulomas with central necrosis (*panel B*). HE stain, magnification 100×. (*Courtesy of* Gregor Gorkiewicz, MD, Institute of Pathology, Medical University of Graz, Graz, Austria.)

hosts are more susceptible to infections with *C difficile* and have an increased risk for severe manifestations of this infection. The risk depends on the underlying disease, the mode of immunosuppression, and the environment. Hypervirulent *C difficile* strains like BI-NAP1-O27 can cause local epidemics in hospitals and are associated with an increased mortality from CDI.[72] The reported rates of CDI in immunocompromised patients, for example in patients after solid organ transplantation, vary considerably. The incidence of CDI in these patients is, however, higher than in the normal population. The rate of CDI was 31% in recipients of lung transplants, about 4% in recipients of kidney transplants, 8% to 15% in recipients of kidney/pancreas transplants, and 3% in liver transplants.[73] About 9% of patients after high-dose chemotherapy and autologous hematopoietic stem cell transplantation developed CDI.[74] Because of frequent hospitalization and exposure to antibiotics, *C difficile* has been reported to be the most common bacterial pathogen causing infectious diarrhea in HIV-infected patients.[45,75] Data on severity and recurrence of CDI in immunocompromised patients are inconclusive. In patients who had solid organ transplantation, there was no increased rate of complicated colitis or relapsing CDI as compared with patients who did not receive a transplant.[73] However, the use of glucocorticoids was associated with an increased mortality in CDI[76] and also an increased rate of relapsing CDI.[73]

For many years, diagnosis for *C difficile* was routinely established using enzyme immunoassays for toxin A and/or toxin B. Although these assays provide results within a short time period and are easy to use, the sensitivity (70%–80%) for diagnosis of CDI is not as good as it has been previously assumed. The assay for the common antigen of *C difficile* is more sensitive; however, it also detects toxin-negative *C difficile* strains not causing disease.[77] Currently, the toxigenic anaerobic culture seems to be the gold standard for diagnosis of CDI; however, it takes up to 72 hours to obtain a result. Recently, real-time PCR assays for the toxin genes of *C difficile* (tcd B, tcd A, tcd C) have been developed for a fast and reliable diagnosis of CDI and they appear to have good sensitivity and specificity.[78]

CDI is treated by antibiotics directed against *C difficile*. Standard therapy is either oral metronidazole (500 mg 3 times a day for 10–14 days) or oral vancomycin (125–250 mg 4 times a day for 10–14 days). In severe forms of CDI or infections with the hypervirulent strain BI-NAP1-O27, vancomycin is superior compared with metronidazole with regard to treatment success and rate of relapses[79]; however, treatment with metronidazole is less expensive and therefore recommended in mild cases. In patients who are immunocompromised, vancomycin should be used as initial therapy. A new nonabsorbable antibiotic fidaxomicin (200 mg twice a day for 10 days) is at least as effective as vancomycin in CDI treatment and has fewer relapse rates.[80] Monoclonal antibodies directed against toxin A and toxin B (single dose of 10 mg/kg body weight intravenously), in addition to antibiotic therapy, also reduce the rate of *C difficile* recurrence.[81]

In recurrent disease, long-term vancomycin therapy (vancomycin pulse and taper) with or without *Saccharomyces boulardii* (500 mg twice a day) or rifaximin (400 mg 3 times a day for 14 days) following a course vancomycin has been shown to be effective.[82] In treatment-refractory cases, the restoration of the altered colonic microbiome by fecal bacteriotherapy (installation of fresh stool of a healthy subject by colonoscopy or enema, "stool transplantation") has been shown to be very effective.[83]

VIRAL INFECTIONS

There are a large number of viruses (eg, astrovirus, picobirnavirus, caliciviruses, adenoviruses) that have been implicated in the etiology of HIV-associated diarrhea.[84]

However, CMV is the most common viral agent in patients with AIDS.[5,85] The risk for developing CMV disease increases when CD4 counts fall below 50 × 10⁹/L and has markedly declined in the era of HAART.[86] CMV colitis is the second most common manifestation of CMV disease, after CMV retinitis, in patients with AIDS.[87] Mild diarrhea in HIV-infected patients may rarely be caused by herpes simplex virus proctocolitis.[88] Herpes simplex virus disease usually manifests as perianal, rectal, or esophageal ulcers causing localized pain but no diarrhea.[89]

Cytomegalovirus (CMV)

Gastrointestinal CMV disease usually occurs among immunocompromised individuals and particularly affects patients with HIV infection, solid organ or hematopoietic stem cell transplantation, or secondary immunodeficiency owing to corticosteroids, immunosuppressive treatment, or chemotherapy.[90–93] Transmission of CMV, a DNA virus and member of the Herpesviridae family, usually occurs by close contact with bodily fluids (ie, urine, saliva, blood, tears, breast milk, vaginal fluids).[94] It is clinically important to differentiate between CMV infection, referring to the detection of CMV antigens or antibodies without clinical features of tissue damage, and CMV disease, where CMV reactivation causes tissue damage with subsequent clinical symptoms.[94,95] Because gastrointestinal CMV disease is a major cause of morbidity and mortality in immunocompromised patients, diagnosis at an early stage is essential and may be best confirmed by endoscopic biopsy and subsequent histologic analysis, including immunologic staining.[90,91,96] Gastrointestinal CMV disease may affect any portion of the gastrointestinal tract, but usually presents as colitis with symptoms ranging from low-grade fever, weight loss, anorexia, and abdominal pain to bloody diarrhea. Fulminant colitis may occur as one of the most severe clinical afflictions.[97] Colonoscopy is the preferred method to establish diagnosis.[69] Endoscopic findings include patchy erythema, edema, erosions, and ulcerations.[98,99]

The role of CMV in exacerbation of inflammatory bowel disease remains unclear. It is currently not established whether CMV worsens inflammation or merely is a surrogate marker for severe colitis.[94] Because most patients with inflammatory bowel disease (IBD) are seropositive for CMV infection and have impaired natural killer cell activity and defects in mucosal immunity, CMV reactivation is a probable event during periods of intestinal inflammation.[94,100,101] Moreover, immunosuppressive drugs enhance susceptibility to CMV reactivation.[94] In patients with severe and/or steroid-refractory ulcerative colitis, local reactivation of CMV can be detected in approximately 30% of the cases, whereas CMV colitis rarely occurs in patients with Crohn disease or mild to moderate ulcerative colitis.[94,102–107] Although one would expect worse prognosis in patients with steroid-refractive ulcerative colitis who have been tested positive for CMV, the presence of CMV in the colon of these patients has not been shown to be associated with disease activity, response to medications, or colectomy rate.[102,106,108–110] In summary, local CMV reactivation might be seen as a secondary event in severe steroid-refractory colitis and does not seem to influence prognosis.[94] Furthermore, there are insufficient data as to whether antiviral therapy affects colectomy and remission rates[94]; however, clinical recommendations include testing for CMV reactivation via leukocyte PCR or immunohistochemistry on colonic biopsy specimens in patients with severe steroid-refractive colitis as well as antiviral therapy (eg, ganciclovir, foscarnet) if colonic CMV is detected.[94]

The most effective antiviral agents in CMV disease are ganciclovir (5 mg/kg intravenously twice daily for at least 3 weeks), an acyclovir derivate, valganciclovir (900 mg twice a day for at least 3 weeks), an oral analog of ganciclovir, and foscarnet (90 mg/kg intravenously twice daily for 3–6 weeks), a pyrophosphate analog inhibiting viral replication.[8,94,111,112] Ganciclovir is the treatment of choice for CMV colitis, however.[113] Foscarnet has the advantage of being less bone marrow suppressive compared with ganciclovir. The newest agent used for CMV disease (eg, CMV retinitis) is cidofovir (5 mg/kg once weekly for at least 2 weeks), which has to be administered intravenously, as is the case for ganciclovir and foscarnet.[8] To our knowledge, however, there are no clinical studies on the use of cidofovir in CMV colitis.

Norovirus

In addition to common enteric viruses such as adenovirus and rotaviruses,[114–118] norovirus, the most common cause of nonbacterial gastroenteritis worldwide, has been recently identified as an unsuspected cause of prolonged morbidity and mortality after chemotherapy and hematopoietic stem cell transplantation (HSCT).[119,120] Norovirus, typically presenting with sudden onset of vomiting and diarrhea, was shown to cause life-threatening gastroenteritis in HSCT recipients and therefore should be considered as a possible infectious agent in the differential diagnosis of diarrhea in these patients.[119] Three genogroups (I, II, IV) of noroviruses, belonging to the family of the Caliciviridae, are pathogenic for humans.[119] In contrast to immunocompetent hosts, who usually have self-limiting symptoms only for a few days, norovirus infection has been reported to cause prolonged gastroenteritis and severe illness in immunocompromised children after intestinal transplantation or chemotherapy.[121–123] Norovirus infection was furthermore shown to persist in adult renal allograft recipients and may present with or without clinical symptoms.[124] Diagnosis is established from fecal samples by reverse-transcriptase PCR for norovirus RNA. Because no specific treatment is available, therapeutic management mainly includes symptomatic treatment, including intravenous fluid and electrolyte substitution, as well as enteral and total parenteral nutrition in protracted illness.[119,124] Reduction of immunosuppressive medication may be considered in cases with severe symptoms and should be performed with great care.[124] A potential role of treatment with oral human immunoglobulin has been recently suggested.[125]

FUNGAL INFECTIONS
Histoplasmosis

Fungi such as *Candida species* can be frequently isolated from the stool of HIV infected patients.[126] However, their role as a causative agent of HIV-associated diarrhea remains unclear.[5] Disseminated infection with the dimorphic fungus *Histoplasma capsulatum* (Histoplasmosis), the most common endemic mycosis in HIV-infected patients, may affect the gastrointestinal tract of AIDS patients subsequently leading to diarrhea.[127] The risk of developing histoplasmosis as well as the severity of illness increase as the CD4 counts decline.[128,129] Fever and abdominal pain have been reported in approximately 70% of the patients with gastrointestinal histoplasmosis while weight loss and diarrhea have been reported in less than 50%.[130,131] Gastrointestinal histoplasmosis often occurs in association with pulmonary and hepatic histoplasmosis and may affect the ileocaecal region.[132]

The diagnosis of gastrointestinal histoplasmosis should be considered in HIV-infected patients with major complications such as gastrointestinal obstruction or bleeding, perforation, an abdominal mass, hepatosplenomegaly, or gastrointestinal symptoms accompanied by weight loss or fever.[131] Diagnosis is established by stool cultures for fungi, culture of urine, blood, and bowel or other tissue specimens, serum and urine *Histoplasma* antigen testing or histopathologic examination of gastrointestinal tissue specimens.[8,131,133] Treatment options for disseminated histoplasmosis include amphotericin B (3 mg/kg daily for 1–2 weeks) followed by oral itraconazole (200 mg 3 times daily for 3 days followed by 200 mg twice daily for at least 12 months).[134] In HIV-infected patients with CD4 counts less than 150 cells/mm^3 in endemic areas, prophylaxis with itraconazole (200 mg daily) is recommended.[134]

Microsporidiosis

Microsporidia are intracellular microorganisms that have recently been reclassified from protozoa to fungi. They result in emerging infections in patients with AIDS, organ transplant recipients, children, travelers, and elderly people.[135] *Enterocytozoon bieneusi* and *Encephalitozoon intestinalis* are the most important species leading to human infections. Most infections are caused by *E bieneusi*. In approximately half of the patients with AIDS suffering from chronic diarrhea, microsporidia may be identified as the causative organism. The prevalence of infection strongly correlates with decreasing CD4 counts and has markedly declined in the era of HAART. Clinical manifestations of microsporidiosis include chronic watery noninflammatory diarrhea, weight loss, abdominal pain, nausea, vomiting, fever, sclerosing cholangitis, and colitis. Diagnosis of microsporidia from stool samples by light microscopy is challenging because of their small size of 1 to 2 μm.[2] Although time-consuming and labor-intensive, transmission electron microscopic examination on small bowel biopsy specimens to identify the polar filament and other species-specific ultrastructural characters remains the diagnostic gold standard.[136] Additional diagnostic methods are light microscopy–based methods, including histologic stains, such as the modified trichrome stain, nucleic acid-based methods (PCR) from clinical samples (eg, tissue biopsies, stool, duodenal aspirates, urine specimens), antigen-based detection methods (eg, immunofluorescence assays, ELISA), and antibody-based detection methods.[136] The only available antimicrobial treatment is albendazole (400 mg twice daily for 3 weeks), which is effective for *E intestinalis*.[137] Similar to cryptosporidial infection, HAART is the best therapy for microsporidia infection.[8]

NONINFECTIOUS DIARRHEA IN HIV-INFECTED PATIENTS
Idiopathic AIDS Enteropathy

A unique entity called "idiopathic AIDS enteropathy" or "HIV enteropathy" can be diagnosed once identifiable infections as well as other causes of diarrhea have been excluded.[3] Multiple factors, including an increase in inflammation and immune activation, as well as decreases in mucosal repair and regeneration, contribute to AIDS enteropathy. The gut-associated lymphoid tissue has been shown to play an important role as one of the early targets in HIV infection and severe CD4 cell depletion.[138] In the early course of HIV infection, massive and progressive depletion of gastrointestinal effector memory CD4 T-lymphocytes[139] results in failure to maintain the epithelial barrier function of the gut mucosa,[138] subsequently enabling translocation of microbial products, such as lipopolysaccharide, peptidoglycans, and viral genomes. These microbial products lead to activation of the gastrointestinal and systemic immune system through stimulation of the innate immune system via Toll-like receptors; however, the resultant activated T cells are a further target for HIV.[5,140,141] HIV enteropathy usually affects the jejunum and has been described to be associated with villus atrophy and crypt hyperplasia.[3,142,143] In conclusion, "idiopathic AIDS enteropathy" or "HIV enteropathy" has emerged as a pathogen-negative diarrhea and may be seen as the result of undiscovered infectious pathogens, inflammatory changes within the gastrointestinal tract caused by HIV itself, other environmental or infectious agents, as well as a complex interplay among all these factors.[3] This form of enteropathy improves with HAART and increasing CD4 counts.

Drug-induced diarrhea has become increasingly important as a cause of diarrhea in HIV-infected patients in the era of HAART. Diarrhea is a common side effect of HAART and often leads to discontinuation of antiretroviral therapy.[144] Protease inhibitors are the most common agents associated with diarrhea as a side effect.[8,145,146] Besides other undesirable side effects, such as metabolic or cardiovascular complications, protease inhibitors frequently cause gastrointestinal disorders ranging from mucosal erosions to epithelial barrier dysfunction and diarrhea.[147-150] Although antimotility agents, such as loperamide, diphenoxylate, and codeine, as well as adsorbents (eg, bismuth subsalicylate) have been considered to be useful, there is lack of good evidence for symptomatic management of drug-induced diarrhea in HIV-infected patients.[5] Therefore, no specific recommendation can be made.

Other Noninfectious Mechanisms

The neurotropic properties of HIV lead to a generalized autonomic neuropathy,[151] therefore another suggested noninfectious mechanism of HIV-associated diarrhea is rapid intestinal transit owing to damage of the autonomic nervous system.[5] Furthermore, diarrhea may be caused by HIV-associated malignancies, such as non-Hodgkin B-cell lymphoma and Kaposi sarcoma.[7,152-156] Multiple effects of HIV infection (eg, opportunistic infections, HIV itself, HAART) may impair exocrine pancreatic function, which in turn leads to chronic diarrhea via fat malabsorption.[5,157,158]

DIARRHEA AFTER HSCT AND AFTER SOLID ORGAN TRANSPLANTATION

Diarrhea after HSCT is a common and often severe problem in these patients and deserves special differential diagnostic considerations. Besides increased rates of gastrointestinal infections, diarrhea can be the result of mucosal damage caused by the myeloablative conditioning regimen, side effects of drugs, and intestinal GVHD. After allogeneic HSCT, GVHD is the most common cause of diarrhea. In contrast, after solid organ transplantation (SOT), infections predominate, followed by drug-induced diarrhea. In long-term immunosuppressive therapy after SOT, lymphoid malignancies, such as posttransplantation lymphoproliferative diseases leading to chronic diarrhea and weight loss, may develop. GVHD is a rare complication after SOT.

Infectious diarrhea after HSCT was present in 30% of patients in a single-center study.[159] In a previous study in the early 1980s, enteric pathogens were found in 40% of patients after bone marrow transplantation; patients with enteric pathogens had a higher mortality rate.[115] Infectious agents found after HSCT are *C difficile*, adenovirus, rotavirus, norovirus, and coxsackievirus.[115,120,159] In one study, giardiasis was detected in 1 of 169 patients, and bacterial culture for enteric pathogens did not yield a cause of diarrhea in this cohort.[159] The most common cause of infectious diarrhea after HSCT is *C difficile*, which can be found in 9% of patients after autologous HSCT.[74] After SOT, CMV disease and *C difficile* are the most widespread causes of diarrhea.[160] Parasitic and fungal infections are less frequent causes of diarrhea after SOT.

Intestinal GVHD After Allogeneic Stem Cell Transplantation

Intestinal GVHD after allogeneic stem cell transplantation is the most common cause of diarrhea in this patient group. It usually occurs beyond day 15 after transplantation. GVHD is caused by transplanted immune cells from a genetically different donor that recognize the tissue of the recipient as foreign, leading to an immune reaction. In patients who also develop skin rash and abnormal liver function tests, the diagnosis of GVHD is very likely. Intestinal GVHD disease can result in high-volume watery diarrhea, protein-loosing enteropathy, and bloody diarrhea, requiring blood transfusions. Diagnosis of intestinal GVHD is usually established by histologic evaluation of intestinal biopsies. GVHD can involve the small and/or the large intestine. Although a rectal biopsy is performed in most patients as an initial diagnostic test, a recent study demonstrated that intestinal GVHD can be present only in the terminal ileum with sparing of the colon in up to 20% of patients.[161] Endoscopic features depend on the severity of the disease. In mild forms, the mucosa can appear normal or show only mild edema, whereas in moderate cases, edema, erythema, and aphthous lesions are present, and in severe forms, mucosal hemorrhage, erosions, ulcerations, and denudation of the mucosa are observed (**Fig. 2**A).[161] Typical histologic changes for intestinal GVHD include apoptotic bodies of the epithelium, crypt cell necrosis, villous blunting in the small intestine, pericapillary hemorrhage, infiltration by neutrophils and eosinophils, and, in severe forms, complete denudation of the epithelium (see **Fig. 2**B).[162] Intestinal GVHD is primarily treated by glucocorticoids, such as methylprednisolone (depending on severity 2–20 mg/kg body weight per day, with subsequent tapering after 5 days) and prednisolone. Second-line treatments include cyclosporine (initially 3–5 mg/kg intravenous; 10–15 mg/kg peroral), antithymocyte globulin (2.5 mg/kg given on alternate days for 6 doses), budesonide (9 mg per day) and TNF blocking agents (infiximab 10 mg/kg intravenously weekly for 4 weeks) or a combination of these agents.[163]

Intestinal GVHD After Autologous Stem Cell Transplantation, SOT, and Blood Transfusion

A clinically and histologically similar syndrome is observed also after autologous stem cell transplantation. The pathophysiology of this syndrome is poorly understood. In a series of 681 patients with autologous stem cell transplantation, the frequency of intestinal GVHD was 13%.[164] This form of GVHD usually responds well to a short course of steroids (prednisone initial dose of 0.5–2.0 mg/kg/d, tapering dependent on response).[164]

In SOT, GVHD is a rare complication. It has been observed in 6% of patients with small intestinal and in 1% to 2% of patients with liver transplantation, but is also

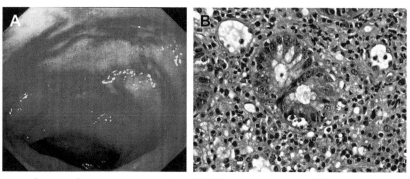

Fig. 2. Endoscopy demonstrating intestinal GVHD. *Panel A* depicts diffuse colitis with irregular shaped ulcers in the right colon. Obtained biopsy of the colon showed histopathological features characteristic of acute GVHD with presence of apoptotic bodies at the crypt basis (*panel B*). HE stain, magnification 400×. (*Courtesy of* Gregor Gorkiewicz, MD, Institute of Pathology, Medical University of Graz, Graz, Austria.)

reported in isolated cases after kidney, pancreas, heart, or lung transplantation.[165] The development of SOT-GVHD is assumed to be related to the solid organ graft containing immunologically competent cells that are activated by alloantigens of the host tissue. As in GVHD owing to other causes, the intestine may be involved, leading to diarrhea, abdominal pain, and gastrointestinal bleeding. The mortality of SOT-GVHD is high and ranges from 30% to 75%.[165]

Transfusion-associated GVHD (TA-GVHD) can occur after transfusion of red blood cells containing also leukocytes. The risk for developing TA-GVHD is highest in recipients with immunodeficiency and in immunocompetent hosts receiving blood donation from relatives. Intestinal involvement in TA-GVHD can lead to high-volume diarrhea and involvement of the small and large intestine.[166] Mortality of TA-GVHD approaches 100%, as it does not respond to medical therapy. Therefore, prevention in immuncompromised patients by irradiation of cellular blood products is essential.

Neutropenic Enterocolitis

Neutropenic enterocolitis is a syndrome in neutropenic patients characterized by abdominal pain and fever. It is mainly observed in patients after chemotherapy, but can also develop in other conditions associated with neutropenia (absolute neutrophil count <500 µg). The incidence is about 5% in patients receiving high-dose chemotherapy for solid tumors and in patients with hematological malignancies.[167] The pathogenesis of the syndrome is not well established; mucosal damage owing to chemotherapeutic agents is suspected, which in turn leads to bacterial infiltration of the bowel wall and necrosis. Inflammation is nearly always present in the cecum. The terminal ileum, other parts of the small intestine, and the colon can be involved.[168] The pain is usually located in the right lower quadrant and diarrhea with or without blood is commonly present. Mortality rate is high and patients die from sepsis or bowel perforation. The diagnosis has to be considered in patients in whom CT scan or ultrasound show thickening and dilatation of the inflamed cecum and other involved intestinal segments.[168] Patients without complications should be managed conservatively, including broad-spectrum antibiotic therapy, total parenteral nutrition, and recombinant granulocyte colony-stimulating factor. Surgery with right hemicolectomy should be performed only in patients with complications such as perforation or bleeding with failure to conservative treatment.[168]

Cord Colitis Syndrome

Herrera and colleagues[169] have described a cord-colitis syndrome occurring in 11 (11%) of 104 of patients after cord blood HSCT.[169] These patients developed persistent diarrhea after a median time of 131 days (range, 88–314) after cord-blood HSCT. Symptoms include nonbloody watery chronic diarrhea, weight loss, and fever. Histologic features of colitis are distinct from intestinal GVHD and include granulomatous inflammation, neutrophilic infiltration of the epithelium and paneth cell metaplasia. Although crypt epithelial apoptosis can be observed, it is less prominent than in acute GVHD. Patients with cord colitis syndrome respond to antibiotic therapy with a combination of metronidazole and a fluoroquinolone (10–14 days treatment duration). Colitis can recur after therapy; however, it usually responds to a subsequent course of antibiotics.[169]

DRUG-INDUCED DIARRHEA

Diarrhea may be a side effect of immunosuppressive drugs (see **Table 2**). Mycophenolate mofetil (MMF) commonly causes diarrhea and colitis is usually present in these patients. The so-called MMF-colitis may show histologic features similar to GVHD.[170] In diarrhea, the dose of MMF must be decreased or the drug must be discontinued. Diarrhea is also frequently observed with calcineurin inhibitor treatment with cyclosporine A, tacrolimus, and sirolimus.[160]

CONGENITAL IMMUNODEFICIENCY SYNDROMES

Diarrhea commonly occurs in different entities that are characterized by deficiencies in humoral or cellular immunity.[171] The immunodeficiency syndromes most commonly associated with diarrhea are selective immunoglobulin (Ig) A deficiency, common variable immunodeficiency (CVID), and severe combined immunodeficiency. The etiology of the diarrhea varies for the different syndromes.

IgA Deficiency

Selective IgA deficiency is the most common primary immunodeficiency disorder and is characterized by a selective near-absence of secretory and serum IgA, leading to susceptibility to respiratory, urogenital, and gastrointestinal infections. Autoimmune and allergic diseases also commonly develop in patients with this disorder. A 10-fold to 16-fold increase in the incidence of gluten-sensitive enteropathy in patients with IgA deficiency has been reported[172]; however, at least a subgroup of patients have sprue-like small intestinal lesions, leading to severe diarrhea and malabsorption, which are unresponsive to a gluten-free diet.[173] Improvement with immunosuppressive therapy has been described in one case report.[174] Giardiasis, and secondary disaccharidase deficiencies leading to diarrhea also are seen with increased frequency in persons with selective IgA deficiency.[173,175]

CVID

Common variable immunodeficiency, or CVID-acquired hypogammaglobulinemia, is an immunodeficiency disorder characterized by decreased serum IgG levels, decreased serum levels of other immunoglobulin subclasses, and T-cell defects. Familial and sporadic forms are caused by mutations in the TNFRSF13B gene.[176] Onset of the disease usually is in adulthood, with recurrent respiratory and gastrointestinal infections. Affected patients also are at increased risk for autoimmune and neoplastic diseases. Malabsorption and diarrhea occur in 9% to 40% of patients with CVID.[173] Small intestinal biopsy specimens show either sprue-like features, including villous shortening with increased numbers of lymphocytes in the epithelium and in the lamina propria, or a pattern similar to that in GVHD.[173,177] Some specific histologic features, namely, a near-absence of plasma cells, are observed. Patients do not respond to a gluten-free diet, and it appears that the sprue-like syndrome in CVID is a distinct entity,[178] sometimes referred to as "hypogammaglobulinemic sprue."[179] In some patients with CVID, foamy macrophages are present, as in Whipple disease, but in contrast to Whipple disease, the macrophages do not contain periodic acid-Schiff–positive material.[177] In addition, nodular lymphoid hyperplasia can be detected in the gastrointestinal tract in a high proportion of patients with CVID; however, the presence of nodular lymphoid hyperplasia does not correlate with the presence of malabsorption or diarrhea. Because the incidence of small bowel lymphoma is increased in CVID, this disorder also has to be considered as a potential cause of diarrhea and malabsorption in these patients. *Giardia* organisms often are isolated from patients with CVID, and small bowel bacterial overgrowth frequently is present. Unfortunately, only some of these patients respond to antimicrobial treatment.[177] Some patients with sprue-like intestinal changes have benefited from glucocorticoids[175] or immunoglobulins.

Other Congenital Immunodeficiency Syndromes

X-linked infantile agammaglobulinemia (Bruton agammaglobulinemia) is caused by mutations in the gene for Bruton tyrosine kinase.[180] This disease usually manifests itself after the first 6 months of life and is characterized by recurrent severe bacterial infections. Severe gastrointestinal problems seem to be less common than in CVID.[177] The prevalence of chronic gastroenteritis was 10% in one large series.[181] In affected patients, giardiasis and bacterial overgrowth need to be considered.[177,181]

Immune dysregulation–polyendocrinopathy–enteropathy–X-linked syndrome (IPEX) is a disorder of early childhood, characterized by protracted diarrhea, dermatitis, insulin-dependent diabetes mellitus, thyroiditis, thrombocytopenia and hemolytic anemia. It is a disorder of X-linked recessive inheritance caused by mutations in the FOXP3 gene.[182] Diarrhea and malabsorption are secondary to severe villus atrophy with inflammation. Antienterocyte antibodies commonly are present. The enteropathy usually does not respond to a gluten-free diet, but immunosuppressive therapy has been shown to be of some benefit. IPEX usually is lethal in childhood. Successful bone marrow transplantation with amelioration of enteropathy has been reported in some cases.[183]

In severe combined immunodeficiency, diarrhea and malabsorption are common. Symptoms are associated with stunting of intestinal villi or their complete absence. The pathophysiology of malabsorption is unknown, and the syndrome usually fails to respond to antimicrobial treatment.[173,175] Chronic granulomatous disease is a genetically heterogeneous immunodeficiency disorder resulting from an inability of phagocytes to destroy microbes. Diarrhea can occur owing to chronic recurrent colitis, which is found in 10% to 30% of patients and shows some histologic features similar to Crohn disease.[184] Diarrhea also has been reported in DiGeorge syndrome (thymic hypoplasia), but little is known about its etiology.[173]

REFERENCES

1. Knox TA, Spiegelman D, Skinner SC, et al. Diarrhea and abnormalities of gastro-intestinal function in a cohort of men and women with HIV infection. Am J Gastroenterol 2000;95:3482–9.
2. Kartalija M, Sande MA. Diarrhea and AIDS in the era of highly active antiretroviral therapy. Clin Infect Dis 1999;28:701–5.
3. Cello JP, Day LW. Idiopathic AIDS enteropathy and treatment of gastrointestinal opportunistic pathogens. Gastroenterology 2009;136:1952–65.
4. Katabira ET. Epidemiology and management of diarrheal disease in HIV-infected patients. Int J Infect Dis 1999;3:164–7.
5. Feasey NA, Healey P, Gordon MA. Review article: the aetiology, investigation and management of diarrhoea in the HIV-positive patient. Aliment Pharmacol Ther 2011;34:587–603.
6. Antony MA, Brandt LJ, Klein RS, et al. Infectious diarrhea in patients with AIDS. Dig Dis Sci 1988;33:1141–6.
7. Connolly GM, Shanson D, Hawkins DA, et al. Non-cryptosporidial diarrhoea in human immunodeficiency virus (HIV) infected patients. Gut 1989;30:195–200.
8. Wilcox CM. Gastrointestinal consequences of infection with human immunodeficiency virus. In: Feldman M, Friedman LS, Brandt LJ, editors. Sleisenger and

Fordtrans's Gastrointestinal and Liver Disease. vol. 1. Philadelphia: Elsevier Saunders; 2010. p. 526–30.

9. Kearney DJ, Steuerwald M, Koch J, et al. A prospective study of endoscopy in HIV-associated diarrhea. Am J Gastroenterol 1999;94:596–602.

10. Thom K, Forrest G. Gastrointestinal infections in immunocompromised hosts. Curr Opin Gastroenterol 2006;22:18–23.

11. Forrest G. Gastrointestinal infections in immunocompromised hosts. Curr Opin Gastroenterol 2004;20:16–21.

12. Fantry L. Gastrointestinal infections in the immunocompromised host. Curr Opin Gastroenterol 2000;16:45–50.

13. Huston CD. Intestinal protozoa. In: Feldman M, Friedman LS, Brandt LJ, editors. Sleisenger and Fordtrans's Gastrointestinal and Liver Disease. vol. 2. Philadelphia: Elsevier Saunders; 2010. p. 1914–8.

14. Caccio SM. Molecular epidemiology of human cryptosporidiosis. Parassitologia 2005;47:185–92.

15. Abubakar I, Aliyu SH, Arumugam C, et al. Treatment of cryptosporidiosis in immunocompromised individuals: systematic review and meta-analysis. Br J Clin Pharmacol 2007;63:387–93.

16. Hunter PR, Nichols G. Epidemiology and clinical features of *Cryptosporidium* infection in immunocompromised patients. Clin Microbiol Rev 2002;15:145–54.

17. Current WL, Garcia LS. Cryptosporidiosis. Clin Microbiol Rev 1991;4:325–58.

18. Deng M, Rutherford MS, Abrahamsen MS. Host intestinal epithelial response to *Cryptosporidium parvum*. Adv Drug Deliv Rev 2004;56:869–84.

19. Ma P. Cryptosporidiosis and immune enteropathy: a review. Curr Clin Top Infect Dis 1987;8:99–153.

20. Colford JM Jr, Tager IB, Hirozawa AM, et al. Cryptosporidiosis among patients infected with human immunodeficiency virus. Factors related to symptomatic infection and survival. Am J Epidemiol 1996;144:807–16.

21. Mwachari C, Batchelor BI, Paul J, et al. Chronic diarrhoea among HIV-infected adult patients in Nairobi, Kenya. J Infect 1998;37:48–53.

22. Ives NJ, Gazzard BG, Easterbrook PJ. The changing pattern of AIDS-defining illnesses with the introduction of highly active antiretroviral therapy (HAART) in a London clinic. J Infect 2001;42:134–9.

23. Miao YM, Awad-El-Kariem FM, Franzen C, et al. Eradication of cryptosporidia and microsporidia following successful antiretroviral therapy. J Acquir Immune Defic Syndr 2000;25:124–9.

24. Cama VA, Ross JM, Crawford S, et al. Differences in clinical manifestations among *Cryptosporidium* species and subtypes in HIV-infected persons. J Infect Dis 2007;196:684–91.

25. Zardi EM, Picardi A, Afeltra A. Treatment of cryptosporidiosis in immunocompromised hosts. Chemotherapy 2005;51:193–6.

26. Silva CV, Ferreira MS, Borges AS, et al. Intestinal parasitic infections in HIV/AIDS patients: experience at a teaching hospital in central Brazil. Scand J Infect Dis 2005;37:211–5.

27. Smith HV, Corcoran GD. New drugs and treatment for cryptosporidiosis. Curr Opin Infect Dis 2004;17:557–64.

28. Rossignol JF. Nitazoxanide in the treatment of acquired immune deficiency syndrome-related cryptosporidiosis: results of the United States compassionate use program in 365 patients. Aliment Pharmacol Ther 2006;24:887–94.

29. Concha R, Harrington W Jr, Rogers AI. Intestinal strongyloidiasis: recognition, management, and determinants of outcome. J Clin Gastroenterol 2005;39:203–11.

30. Abrescia FF, Falda A, Caramaschi G, et al. Reemergence of strongyloidiasis, northern Italy. Emerg Infect Dis 2009;15:1531–3.
31. Ganesh S, Cruz RJ Jr. Strongyloidiasis: a multifaceted disease. Gastroenterol Hepatol (N Y) 2011;7:194–6.
32. Segarra-Newnham M. Manifestations, diagnosis, and treatment of Strongyloides stercoralis infection. Ann Pharmacother 2007;41:1992–2001.
33. Siddiqui AA, Berk SL. Diagnosis of Strongyloides stercoralis infection. Clin Infect Dis 2001;33:1040–7.
34. Mahmoud AA. Strongyloidiasis. Clin Infect Dis 1996;23:949–52.
35. Kakati B, Dang S, Heif M, et al. Strongyloides duodenitis: case report and review of literature. J Natl Med Assoc 2011;103:60–3.
36. Keiser PB, Nutman TB. Strongyloides stercoralis in the immunocompromised population. Clin Microbiol Rev 2004;17:208–17.
37. Montes M, Sawhney C, Barros N. Strongyloides stercoralis: there but not seen. Curr Opin Infect Dis 2010;23:500–4.
38. Ackers JP. Gut coccidia–isospora, cryptosporidium, cyclospora and sarcocystis. Semin Gastrointest Dis 1997;8:33–44.
39. Guk SM, Seo M, Park YK, et al. Parasitic infections in HIV-infected patients who visited Seoul National University Hospital during the period 1995-2003. Korean J Parasitol 2005;43:1–5.
40. Atambay M, Bayraktar MR, Kayabas U, et al. A rare diarrheic parasite in a liver transplant patient: Isospora belli. Transplant Proc 2007;39:1693–5.
41. Yazar S, Tokgoz B, Yaman O, et al. Isospora belli infection in a patient with a renal transplant. Turkiye Parazitol Derg 2006;30:22–4 [in Turkish].
42. Koru O, Araz RE, Yilmaz YA, et al. Case report: Isospora belli infection in a renal transplant recipient. Turkiye Parazitol Derg 2007;31:98–100.
43. Pape JW, Verdier RI, Johnson WD Jr. Treatment and prophylaxis of Isospora belli infection in patients with the acquired immunodeficiency syndrome. N Engl J Med 1989;320:1044–7.
44. Verdier RI, Fitzgerald DW, Johnson WD Jr, et al. Trimethoprim-sulfamethoxazole compared with ciprofloxacin for treatment and prophylaxis of Isospora belli and Cyclospora cayetanensis infection in HIV-infected patients. A randomized, controlled trial. Ann Intern Med 2000;132:885–8.
45. Sanchez TH, Brooks JT, Sullivan PS, et al. Bacterial diarrhea in persons with HIV infection, United States, 1992-2002. Clin Infect Dis 2005;41:1621–7.
46. Fernandez-Cruz A, Munoz P, Mohedano R, et al. Campylobacter bacteremia: clinical characteristics, incidence, and outcome over 23 years. Medicine (Baltimore) 2010;89:319–30.
47. Pigrau C, Almirante B, Bartolome R, et al. Bacteremia due to Campylobacter sp. in patients with HIV infection. Med Clin (Barc) 1994;103:239 [in Spanish].
48. Hsu RB, Lin FY. Nontyphoid Salmonella infection in heart transplant recipients. Am J Med Sci 2008;336:393–6.
49. Hohmann EL. Nontyphoidal salmonellosis. Clin Infect Dis 2001;32:263–9.
50. Ramos JM, Garcia-Corbeira P, Aguado JM, et al. Nontyphoid Salmonella extraintestinal infections in renal transplant recipients. Nephron 1995;71:489–90.
51. Huang JY, Huang CC, Lai MK, et al. Salmonella infection in renal transplant recipients. Transplant Proc 1994;26:2147.
52. Dhar JM, al-Khader AA, al-Sulaiman M, et al. Non-typhoid Salmonella in renal transplant recipients: a report of twenty cases and review of the literature. Q J Med 1991;78:235–50.

53. Ejlertsen T, Aunsholt NA. Salmonella bacteremia in renal transplant recipients. Scand J Infect Dis 1989;21:241–4.
54. Ocharan-Corcuera J, Montejo-Baranda M, Lampreabe-Gaztelu I, et al. Nontyphoid Salmonella infections after renal transplantation. Transplantation 1987; 44:150–1.
55. Samra Y, Shaked Y, Maier MK. Nontyphoid salmonellosis in renal transplant recipients: report of five cases and review of the literature. Rev Infect Dis 1986;8:431–40.
56. de la Monte SM, Hutchins GM. Follicular proctocolitis and neuromatous hyperplasia with lymphogranuloma venereum. Hum Pathol 1985;16:1025–32.
57. van Nieuwkoop C, Gooskens J, Smit VT, et al. Lymphogranuloma venereum proctocolitis: mucosal T cell immunity of the rectum associated with chlamydial clearance and clinical recovery. Gut 2007;56:1476–7.
58. Burgers WA, Riou C, Mlotshwa M, et al. Association of HIV-specific and total CD8 + T memory phenotypes in subtype C HIV-1 infection with viral set point. J Immunol 2009;182:4751–61.
59. Horsburgh CR Jr. Mycobacterium avium complex infection in the acquired immunodeficiency syndrome. N Engl J Med 1991;324:1332–8.
60. Wallace JM, Hannah JB. Mycobacterium avium complex infection in patients with the acquired immunodeficiency syndrome. A clinicopathologic study. Chest 1988;93:926–32.
61. Hawkins CC, Gold JW, Whimbey E, et al. Mycobacterium avium complex infections in patients with the acquired immunodeficiency syndrome. Ann Intern Med 1986;105:184–8.
62. Horsburgh CR Jr, Selik RM. The epidemiology of disseminated nontuberculous mycobacterial infection in the acquired immunodeficiency syndrome (AIDS). Am Rev Respir Dis 1989;139:4–7.
63. Ellner JJ, Goldberger MJ, Parenti DM. Mycobacterium avium infection and AIDS: a therapeutic dilemma in rapid evolution. J Infect Dis 1991;163:1326–35.
64. Benson CA, Ellner JJ. Mycobacterium avium complex infection and AIDS: advances in theory and practice. Clin Infect Dis 1993;17:7–20.
65. Nightingale SD, Byrd LT, Southern PM, et al. Incidence of Mycobacterium avium-intracellulare complex bacteremia in human immunodeficiency virus-positive patients. J Infect Dis 1992;165:1082–5.
66. Karakousis PC, Moore RD, Chaisson RE. Mycobacterium avium complex in patients with HIV infection in the era of highly active antiretroviral therapy. Lancet Infect Dis 2004;4:557–65.
67. Chaisson RE, Moore RD, Richman DD, et al. Incidence and natural history of Mycobacterium avium-complex infections in patients with advanced human immunodeficiency virus disease treated with zidovudine. The Zidovudine Epidemiology Study Group. Am Rev Respir Dis 1992;146:285–9.
68. Gordin FM, Cohn DL, Sullam PM, et al. Early manifestations of disseminated Mycobacterium avium complex disease: a prospective evaluation. J Infect Dis 1997;176:126–32.
69. Bhaijee F, Subramony C, Tang SJ, et al. Human immunodeficiency virus-associated gastrointestinal disease: common endoscopic biopsy diagnoses. Patholog Res Int 2011;2011:247923.
70. Sun HY, Chen MY, Wu MS, et al. Endoscopic appearance of GI mycobacteriosis caused by the Mycobacterium avium complex in a patient with AIDS: case report and review. Gastrointest Endosc 2005;61:775–9.

71. Loo VG, Bourgault AM, Poirier L, et al. Host and pathogen factors for *Clostridium difficile* infection and colonization. N Engl J Med 2011;365:1693–703.

72. Kelly CP, LaMont JT. *Clostridium difficile*—more difficult than ever. N Engl J Med 2008;359:1932–40.

73. Gellad ZF, Alexander BD, Liu JK, et al. Severity of *Clostridium difficile*-associated diarrhea in solid organ transplant patients. Transpl Infect Dis 2007;9:276–80.

74. Gil L, Styczynski J, Komarnicki M. Infectious complication in 314 patients after high-dose therapy and autologous hematopoietic stem cell transplantation: risk factors analysis and outcome. Infection 2007;35:421–7.

75. Willingham FF, Ticona Chavez E, Taylor DN, et al. Diarrhea and *Clostridium difficile* infection in Latin American patients with AIDS. Working Group on AIDS in Peru. Clin Infect Dis 1998;27:487–93.

76. Das R, Feuerstadt P, Brandt LJ. Glucocorticoids are associated with increased risk of short-term mortality in hospitalized patients with *Clostridium difficile*-associated disease. Am J Gastroenterol 2010;105:2040–9.

77. Bartlett JG, Gerding DN. Clinical recognition and diagnosis of Clostridium difficile infection. Clin Infect Dis 2008;46(Suppl 1):S12–8.

78. Deshpande A, Pasupuleti V, Rolston DD, et al. Diagnostic accuracy of real-time polymerase chain reaction in detection of *Clostridium difficile* in the stool samples of patients with suspected *Clostridium difficile* infection: a meta-analysis. Clin Infect Dis 2011;53:e81–90.

79. Zar FA, Bakkanagari SR, Moorthi KM, et al. A comparison of vancomycin and metronidazole for the treatment of *Clostridium difficile*-associated diarrhea, stratified by disease severity. Clin Infect Dis 2007;45:302–7.

80. Louie TJ, Miller MA, Mullane KM, et al. Fidaxomicin versus vancomycin for *Clostridium difficile* infection. N Engl J Med 2011;364:422–31.

81. Lowy I, Molrine DC, Leav BA, et al. Treatment with monoclonal antibodies against *Clostridium difficile* toxins. N Engl J Med 2010;362:197–205.

82. Bauer MP, Kuijper EJ, van Dissel JT. European Society of Clinical Microbiology and Infectious Diseases (ESCMID): treatment guidance document for *Clostridium difficile* infection (CDI). Clin Microbiol Infect 2009;15:1067–79.

83. Landy J, Al-Hassi HO, McLaughlin SD, et al. Review article: faecal transplantation therapy for gastrointestinal disease. Aliment Pharmacol Ther 2011;34:409–15.

84. Grohmann GS, Glass RI, Pereira HG, et al. Enteric viruses and diarrhea in HIV-infected patients. Enteric Opportunistic Infections Working Group. N Engl J Med 1993;329:14–20.

85. Gertler SL, Pressman J, Price P, et al. Gastrointestinal cytomegalovirus infection in a homosexual man with severe acquired immunodeficiency syndrome. Gastroenterology 1983;85:1403–6.

86. Salzberger B, Hartmann P, Hanses F, et al. Incidence and prognosis of CMV disease in HIV-infected patients before and after introduction of combination antiretroviral therapy. Infection 2005;33:345–9.

87. Jacobson MA, Mills J. Serious cytomegalovirus disease in the acquired immunodeficiency syndrome (AIDS). Clinical findings, diagnosis, and treatment. Ann Intern Med 1988;108:585–94.

88. Smith PD, Lane HC, Gill VJ, et al. Intestinal infections in patients with the acquired immunodeficiency syndrome (AIDS). Etiology and response to therapy. Ann Intern Med 1988;108:328–33.

89. Sinicco A, Palestro G, Caramello P, et al. Acute HIV-1 infection: clinical and biological study of 12 patients. J Acquir Immune Defic Syndr 1990;3:260–5.

90. Baroco AL, Oldfield EC. Gastrointestinal cytomegalovirus disease in the immunocompromised patient. Curr Gastroenterol Rep 2008;10:409–16.
91. Goodgame RW. Gastrointestinal cytomegalovirus disease. Ann Intern Med 1993;119:924–35.
92. Mori T, Mori S, Kanda Y, et al. Clinical significance of cytomegalovirus (CMV) antigenemia in the prediction and diagnosis of CMV gastrointestinal disease after allogeneic hematopoietic stem cell transplantation. Bone Marrow Transplant 2004;33:431–4.
93. Fujita M, Hatachi S, Yagita M. Immunohistochemically proven cytomegalovirus gastrointestinal diseases in three patients with autoimmune diseases. Clin Rheumatol 2008;27:1057–9.
94. Lawlor G, Moss AC. Cytomegalovirus in inflammatory bowel disease: pathogen or innocent bystander? Inflamm Bowel Dis 2010;16:1620–7.
95. Ayre K, Warren BF, Jeffery K, et al. The role of CMV in steroid-resistant ulcerative colitis: a systematic review. J Crohns Colitis 2009;3:141–8.
96. Drew WL. Diagnosis of cytomegalovirus infection. Rev Infect Dis 1988;10(Suppl 3): S468–76.
97. Dieterich DT, Rahmin M. Cytomegalovirus colitis in AIDS: presentation in 44 patients and a review of the literature. J Acquir Immune Defic Syndr 1991; 4(Suppl 1):S29–35.
98. Rene E, Marche C, Chevalier T, et al. Cytomegalovirus colitis in patients with acquired immunodeficiency syndrome. Dig Dis Sci 1988;33:741–50.
99. Ljungman P, Griffiths P, Paya C. Definitions of cytomegalovirus infection and disease in transplant recipients. Clin Infect Dis 2002;34:1094–7.
100. Targan SR, Karp LC. Defects in mucosal immunity leading to ulcerative colitis. Immunol Rev 2005;206:296–305.
101. Ginsburg CH, Dambrauskas JT, Ault KA, et al. Impaired natural killer cell activity in patients with inflammatory bowel disease: evidence for a qualitative defect. Gastroenterology 1983;85:846–51.
102. Kambham N, Vij R, Cartwright CA, et al. Cytomegalovirus infection in steroid-refractory ulcerative colitis: a case-control study. Am J Surg Pathol 2004;28: 365–73.
103. Orvar K, Murray J, Carmen G, et al. Cytomegalovirus infection associated with onset of inflammatory bowel disease. Dig Dis Sci 1993;38:2307–10.
104. Knosel T, Schewe C, Petersen N, et al. Prevalence of infectious pathogens in Crohn's disease. Pathol Res Pract 2009;205:223–30.
105. Cottone M, Pietrosi G, Martorana G, et al. Prevalence of cytomegalovirus infection in severe refractory ulcerative and Crohn's colitis. Am J Gastroenterol 2001; 96:773–5.
106. Domenech E, Vega R, Ojanguren I, et al. Cytomegalovirus infection in ulcerative colitis: a prospective, comparative study on prevalence and diagnostic strategy. Inflamm Bowel Dis 2008;14:1373–9.
107. Maconi G, Colombo E, Zerbi P, et al. Prevalence, detection rate and outcome of cytomegalovirus infection in ulcerative colitis patients requiring colonic resection. Dig Liver Dis 2005;37:418–23.
108. Kojima T, Watanabe T, Hata K, et al. Cytomegalovirus infection in ulcerative colitis. Scand J Gastroenterol 2006;41:706–11.
109. Matsuoka K, Iwao Y, Mori T, et al. Cytomegalovirus is frequently reactivated and disappears without antiviral agents in ulcerative colitis patients. Am J Gastroenterol 2007;102:331–7.

110. Yoshino T, Nakase H, Ueno S, et al. Usefulness of quantitative real-time PCR assay for early detection of cytomegalovirus infection in patients with ulcerative colitis refractory to immunosuppressive therapies. Inflamm Bowel Dis 2007;13: 1516–21.

111. Markham A, Faulds D. Ganciclovir. An update of its therapeutic use in cytomeg-alovirus infection. Drugs 1994;48:455–84.

112. Faulds D, Heel RC. Ganciclovir. A review of its antiviral activity, pharmacokinetic properties and therapeutic efficacy in cytomegalovirus infections. Drugs 1990; 39:597–638.

113. Kandiel A, Lashner B. Cytomegalovirus colitis complicating inflammatory bowel disease. Am J Gastroenterol 2006;101:2857–65.

114. van Kraaij MG, Dekker AW, Verdonck LF, et al. Infectious gastro-enteritis: an uncommon cause of diarrhoea in adult allogeneic and autologous stem cell transplant recipients. Bone Marrow Transplant 2000;26:299–303.

115. Yolken RH, Bishop CA, Townsend TR, et al. Infectious gastroenteritis in bone-marrow-transplant recipients. N Engl J Med 1982;306:1010–2.

116. Cox GJ, Matsui SM, Lo RS, et al. Etiology and outcome of diarrhea after marrow transplantation: a prospective study. Gastroenterology 1994;107:1398–407.

117. Troussard X, Bauduer F, Gallet E, et al. Virus recovery from stools of patients under-going bone marrow transplantation. Bone Marrow Transplant 1993;12:573–6.

118. Yuen KY, Woo PC, Liang RH, et al. Clinical significance of alimentary tract microbes in bone marrow transplant recipients. Diagn Microbiol Infect Dis 1998;30:75–81.

119. Roddie C, Paul JP, Benjamin R, et al. Allogeneic hematopoietic stem cell trans-plantation and norovirus gastroenteritis: a previously unrecognized cause of morbidity. Clin Infect Dis 2009;49:1061–8.

120. Schwartz S, Vergoulidou M, Schreier E, et al. Norovirus gastroenteritis causes severe and lethal complications after chemotherapy and hematopoietic stem cell transplantation. Blood 2011;117:5850–6.

121. Kaufman SS, Chatterjee NK, Fuschino ME, et al. Characteristics of human cal-icivirus enteritis in intestinal transplant recipients. J Pediatr Gastroenterol Nutr 2005;40:328–33.

122. Ludwig A, Adams O, Laws HJ, et al. Quantitative detection of norovirus excre-tion in pediatric patients with cancer and prolonged gastroenteritis and shed-ding of norovirus. J Med Virol 2008;80:1461–7.

123. Simon A, Schildgen O, Maria Eis-Hubinger A, et al. Norovirus outbreak in a pedi-atric oncology unit. Scand J Gastroenterol 2006;41:693–9.

124. Schorn R, Hohne M, Meerbach A, et al. Chronic norovirus infection after kidney transplantation: molecular evidence for immune-driven viral evolution. Clin Infect Dis 2010;51:307–14.

125. Florescu DF, Hermsen ED, Kwon JY, et al. Is there a role for oral human immu-noglobulin in the treatment for norovirus enteritis in immunocompromised patients? Pediatr Transplant 2011;15:718–21.

126. Uppal B, Kashyap B, Bhalla P. Enteric pathogens in HIV/AIDS from a tertiary care hospital. Indian J Community Med 2009;34:237–42.

127. Casotti JA, Motta TQ, Ferreira CU Jr, et al. Disseminated histoplasmosis in HIV positive patients in Espirito Santo state, Brazil: a clinical-laboratory study of 12 cases (1999-2001). Braz J Infect Dis 2006;10:327–30.

128. Wheat LJ, Connolly-Stringfield PA, Baker RL, et al. Disseminated histoplasmosis in the acquired immune deficiency syndrome: clinical findings, diagnosis and treatment, and review of the literature. Medicine (Baltimore) 1990;69:361–74.

129. Wheat J. Endemic mycoses in AIDS: a clinical review. Clin Microbiol Rev 1995;8: 146–59.
130. Kahi CJ, Wheat LJ, Allen SD, et al. Gastrointestinal histoplasmosis. Am J Gastroenterol 2005;100:220–31.
131. Suh KN, Anekthananon T, Mariuz PR. Gastrointestinal histoplasmosis in patients with AIDS: case report and review. Clin Infect Dis 2001;32:483–91.
132. Becherer PR, Sokol-Anderson M, Joist JH, et al. Gastrointestinal histoplasmosis presenting as hematochezia in human immunodeficiency virus-infected hemophilic patients. Am J Hematol 1994;47:229–31.
133. Assi M, McKinsey DS, Driks MR, et al. Gastrointestinal histoplasmosis in the acquired immunodeficiency syndrome: report of 18 cases and literature review. Diagn Microbiol Infect Dis 2006;55:195–201.
134. Wheat LJ, Freifeld AG, Kleiman MB, et al. Clinical practice guidelines for the management of patients with histoplasmosis: 2007 update by the Infectious Diseases Society of America. Clin Infect Dis 2007;45:807–25.
135. Anane S, Attouchi H. Microsporidiosis: epidemiology, clinical data and therapy. Gastroenterol Clin Biol 2010;34:450–64.
136. Ghosh K, Weiss LM. Molecular diagnostic tests for microsporidia. Interdiscip Perspect Infect Dis 2009;2009:926521.
137. Molina JM, Chastang C, Goguel J, et al. Albendazole for treatment and prophylaxis of microsporidiosis due to *Encephalitozoon intestinalis* in patients with AIDS: a randomized double-blind controlled trial. J Infect Dis 1998;177: 1373–7.
138. Sankaran S, George MD, Reay E, et al. Rapid onset of intestinal epithelial barrier dysfunction in primary human immunodeficiency virus infection is driven by an imbalance between immune response and mucosal repair and regeneration. J Virol 2008;82:538–45.
139. Veazey RS, DeMaria M, Chalifoux LV, et al. Gastrointestinal tract as a major site of CD4 + T cell depletion and viral replication in SIV infection. Science 1998;280: 427–31.
140. Gordon SN, Cervasi B, Odorizzi P, et al. Disruption of intestinal CD4 + T cell homeostasis is a key marker of systemic CD4 + T cell activation in HIV-infected individuals. J Immunol 2010;185:5169–79.
141. Brenchley JM, Douek DC. HIV infection and the gastrointestinal immune system. Mucosal Immunol 2008;1:23–30.
142. Batman PA, Miller AR, Forster SM, et al. Jejunal enteropathy associated with human immunodeficiency virus infection: quantitative histology. J Clin Pathol 1989;42:275–81.
143. Kotler DP, Gaetz HP, Lange M, et al. Enteropathy associated with the acquired immunodeficiency syndrome. Ann Intern Med 1984;101:421–8.
144. O'Brien ME, Clark RA, Besch CL, et al. Patterns and correlates of discontinuation of the initial HAART regimen in an urban outpatient cohort. J Acquir Immune Defic Syndr 2003;34:407–14.
145. Markowitz M, Saag M, Powderly WG, et al. A preliminary study of ritonavir, an inhibitor of HIV-1 protease, to treat HIV-1 infection. N Engl J Med 1995;333:1534–9.
146. Kempf DJ, Marsh KC, Kumar G, et al. Pharmacokinetic enhancement of inhibitors of the human immunodeficiency virus protease by coadministration with ritonavir. Antimicrob Agents Chemother 1997;41:654–60.
147. Wu X, Sun L, Zha W, et al. HIV protease inhibitors induce endoplasmic reticulum stress and disrupt barrier integrity in intestinal epithelial cells. Gastroenterology 2010;138:197–209.

148. Bode H, Schmidt W, Schulzke JD, et al. Effects of HIV protease inhibitors on barrier function in the human intestinal cell line HT-29/B6. Ann N Y Acad Sci 2000;915:117–22.

149. Bode H, Schmidt W, Schulzke JD, et al. The HIV protease inhibitors saquinavir, ritonavir, and nelfinavir but not indinavir impair the epithelial barrier in the human intestinal cell line HT-29/B6. AIDS 1999;13:2595–7.

150. Bode H, Lenzner L, Kraemer OH, et al. The HIV protease inhibitors saquinavir, ritonavir, and nelfinavir induce apoptosis and decrease barrier function in human intestinal epithelial cells. Antivir Ther 2005;10:645–55.

151. Ruttimann S, Hilti P, Spinas GA, et al. High frequency of human immunodeficiency virus-associated autonomic neuropathy and more severe involvement in advanced stages of human immunodeficiency virus disease. Arch Intern Med 1991;151:2441–3.

152. Dinh MH, Matkowskyj KA, Stosor V. Colorectal lymphoma in the setting of HIV: case report and review of the literature. AIDS Patient Care STDS 2009;23: 227–30.

153. Siani LM, Siani A, Ricci V, et al. Burkitt's lymphoma of the caecum in a patient with AIDS: clinical case and review of the literature. Minerva Chir 2009;64: 229–33 [in Italian].

154. Cappell MS, Botros N. Predominantly gastrointestinal symptoms and signs in 11 consecutive AIDS patients with gastrointestinal lymphoma: a multicenter, multiyear study including 763 HIV-seropositive patients. Am J Gastroenterol 1994;89: 545–9.

155. Kahl P, Buettner R, Friedrichs N, et al. Kaposi's sarcoma of the gastrointestinal tract: report of two cases and review of the literature. Pathol Res Pract 2007;203: 227–31.

156. Lee HF, Lu CL, Chang FY. A man with loose stool and periumbilical pain. Gastroenterology 2010;139(734):1068.

157. Price DA, Schmid ML, Ong EL, et al. Pancreatic exocrine insufficiency in HIV-positive patients. HIV Med 2005;6:33–6.

158. Dassopoulos T, Ehrenpreis ED. Acute pancreatitis in human immunodeficiency virus-infected patients: a review. Am J Med 1999;107:78–84.

159. Kamboj M, Mihu CN, Sepkowitz K, et al. Work-up for infectious diarrhea after allogeneic hematopoietic stem cell transplantation: single specimen testing results in cost savings without compromising diagnostic yield. Transpl Infect Dis 2007;9:265–9.

160. Ginsburg PM, Thuluvath PJ. Diarrhea in liver transplant recipients: etiology and management. Liver Transpl 2005;11:881–90.

161. Kreisel W, Dahlberg M, Bertz H, et al. Endoscopic diagnosis of acute intestinal GVHD following allogeneic hematopoietic SCT: a retrospective analysis in 175 patients. Bone Marrow Transplant 2012;47(3):430–8.

162. Washington K, Jagasia M. Pathology of graft-versus-host disease in the gastrointestinal tract. Hum Pathol 2009;40:909–17.

163. Ferrara JL, Levine JE, Reddy P, et al. Graft-versus-host disease. Lancet 2009; 373:1550–61.

164. Holmberg L, Kikuchi K, Gooley TA, et al. Gastrointestinal graft-versus-host disease in recipients of autologous hematopoietic stem cells: incidence, risk factors, and outcome. Biol Blood Marrow Transplant 2006;12:226–34.

165. Zhang Y, Ruiz P. Solid organ transplant-associated acute graft-versus-host disease. Arch Pathol Lab Med 2010;134:1220–4.

166. Amrein K, Posch U, Langner C, et al. Transfusion-associated graft-versus-host disease presenting as severe high-volume diarrhoea in a patient with Goodpasture's syndrome. Intensive Care Med 2010;36:1271–2.

167. Gorschluter M, Mey U, Strehl J, et al. Neutropenic enterocolitis in adults: systematic analysis of evidence quality. Eur J Haematol 2005;75:1–13.

168. Davila ML. Neutropenic enterocolitis. Curr Opin Gastroenterol 2006;22:44–7.

169. Herrera AF, Soriano G, Bellizzi AM, et al. Cord colitis syndrome in cord-blood stem-cell transplantation. N Engl J Med 2011;365:815–24.

170. Selbst MK, Ahrens WA, Robert ME, et al. Spectrum of histologic changes in colonic biopsies in patients treated with mycophenolate mofetil. Mod Pathol 2009;22:737–43.

171. Spickett GP, Misbah SA, Chapel HM. Primary antibody deficiency in adults. Lancet 1991;337:281–4.

172. Cataldo F, Marino V, Ventura A, et al. Prevalence and clinical features of selective immunoglobulin A deficiency in coeliac disease: an Italian multicentre study. Italian Society of Paediatric Gastroenterology and Hepatology (SIGEP) and "Club del Tenue" Working Groups on Coeliac Disease. Gut 1998;42:362–5.

173. Ament ME. Immunodeficiency syndromes and gastrointestinal disease. Pediatr Clin North Am 1975;22:807–25.

174. McCarthy DM, Katz SI, Gazze L, et al. Selective IgA deficiency associated with total villous atrophy of the small intestine and an organ-specific anti-epithelial cell antibody. J Immunol 1978;120:932–8.

175. Doe WF, Hapel AJ. Intestinal immunity and malabsorption. Clin Gastroenterol 1983;12:415–35.

176. Castigli E, Wilson SA, Garibyan L, et al. TACI is mutant in common variable immunodeficiency and IgA deficiency. Nat Genet 2005;37:829–34.

177. Washington K, Stenzel TT, Buckley RH, et al. Gastrointestinal pathology in patients with common variable immunodeficiency and X-linked agammaglobulinemia. Am J Surg Pathol 1996;20:1240–52.

178. Cunningham-Rundles C. Clinical and immunologic analyses of 103 patients with common variable immunodeficiency. J Clin Immunol 1989;9:22–33.

179. Lewin KJ, Riddell RH, Weinstein WM. Gastrointestinal pathology and its clinical implications. New York: Igaku-Shoin; 1992.

180. Vetrie D, Vorechovsky I, Sideras P, et al. The gene involved in X-linked agammaglobulinaemia is a member of the src family of protein-tyrosine kinases. Nature 1993;361:226–33.

181. Lederman HM, Winkelstein JA. X-linked agammaglobulinemia: an analysis of 96 patients. Medicine (Baltimore) 1985;64:145–56.

182. Bennett CL, Christie J, Ramsdell F, et al. The immune dysregulation, polyendocrinopathy, enteropathy, X-linked syndrome (IPEX) is caused by mutations of FOXP3. Nat Genet 2001;27:20–1.

183. Baud O, Goulet O, Canioni D, et al. Treatment of the immune dysregulation, polyendocrinopathy, enteropathy, X-linked syndrome (IPEX) by allogeneic bone marrow transplantation. N Engl J Med 2001;344:1758–62.

184. Guerrerio AL, Frischmeyer-Guerrerio PA, Lederman HM, et al. Recognizing gastrointestinal and hepatic manifestations of primary immunodeficiency diseases. J Pediatr Gastroenterol Nutr 2010;51:548–55.

Index

Note: Page numbers of article titles are in **boldface** type.

A

Abdominal pain, in lactose malabsorption, 618–619
Acetate, formation of, in carbohydrate metabolism, 612–613
Adalimumab, for microscopic colitis, 658
Agammaglobulinemia, 692
Albendazole
    for microsporidiosis, 687
    for strongyloidiasis, 681
Alosetron, for functional diarrhea, 632
5-Aminosalicylates, for microscopic colitis, 657
Amitriptyline, for functional diarrhea, 632
Amoxicillin, for inflammatory bowel disease, 594–595
Amphotericin B, for histoplasmosis, 687
Ampicillin, carbohydrate metabolism and, 614–615
Anaerobic culture, for *Clostridium difficile,* 684
Anthrone method, for fecal carbohydrates, 622
Antibiotic(s)
    carbohydrate metabolism and, 614–615
    for bacterial overgrowth, 592–593
    for inflammatory bowel disease, 592, 594–595
    for irritable bowel syndrome, 592–593
    gut microbiota alterations by, 585–587
Antibiotic-associated diarrhea, treatment of, 587, 589–590
Antisecretory agents, for functional diarrhea, 634
Antithymocyte globulin, for graft-versus-host disease, 689
AST-120, for functional diarrhea, 633
Atropine, for functional diarrhea, 632
Atypical microscopic colitis, 567–568
Autonomic neuropathy, in HIV infection, 688
Azathioprine
    for inflammatory bowel disease, 594–595
    for microscopic colitis, 657–658
Azithromycin, for mycobacterial infections, 683

B

Bacteremia, *Campylobacter,* 682
Bacterial flora. *See* Gut microbiota.
Bacterial overgrowth, 583–584, 667
    in inflammatory bowel disease, 662–663
    treatment of, 592–593
Bifidobacterium bifidum, for irritable bowel syndrome, 587

Gastroenterol Clin N Am 41 (2012) 703–715
http://dx.doi.org/10.1016/S0889-8553(12)00086-6
0889-8553/12/$ – see front matter © 2012 Elsevier Inc. All rights reserved.

Bifidobacterium breve
   for inflammatory bowel disease, 590
   for irritable bowel syndrome, 587–588
Bifidobacterium infantis, for irritable bowel syndrome, 587–588
Bifidobacterium lactis, for irritable bowel syndrome, 587–588
Bifidobacterium longum, for irritable bowel syndrome, 587–588
Bile acid malabsorption, 660–661
   in inflammatory bowel disease, 666
   in microscopic colitis, 654
Bile-acid binding agents, for functional diarrhea, 633
Biopsy. *See also* Colorectal histopathology.
   for celiac disease, 642–643
   for common variable immunodeficiency, 691
   for graft-versus-host disease, 689
   for microscopic colitis, 655
   for microsporidiosis, 687
   for mycobacterial infections, 683
   for strongyloidiasis, 681
Bismuth subsalicylate
   for functional diarrhea, 633
   for microscopic colitis, 657
Bloating, in lactose malabsorption, 618–619
Blood transfusions, graft-versus-host disease in, 690
Bruton agammaglobulinemia, 692
Budesonide
   for graft-versus-host disease, 689
   for microscopic colitis, 655, 657
Bulking agents
   for functional diarrhea, 633
   for inflammatory bowel disease, 668
Butyrates, formation of, in carbohydrate metabolism, 612–613

C

Calcineurin inhibitors, diarrhea induced by, 691
Calcitonin, in medullary carcinoma of thyroid, 607
Calcium polycarbophil, for inflammatory bowel disease, 668
Campylobacter infections, 682
Carbohydrate malabsorption, **611–627,** 660–662
   antibiotic effects on, 614–615
   causes of, 622–623
   colon absorption in, 613–614
   colonic transit and, 615–616
   definition of, 622
   diagnosis of, 544–547, 552, 554–555, 621–622
   fructose, 619–620
   in disaccharidase deficiencies, 620–621
   in malabsorptive diseases, 616–617
   in Roux-en-Y gastric bypass, 617–618
   lactose, 618–619
   multiple factors in, 616
   organic acid formation and, 623–624

symptoms of, 623
Carcinoid syndrome, 605–606
Celiac disease, **639–650**
    conditions associated with, 644
    definitions of, 639–641
    diagnosis of, 641–643
    diarrhea in, 643–645
    epidemiology of, 639
    latent, 640–641
    nonresponsive, 643
    potential, 641
    refractory, 644–645
Chemotherapy
    for carcinoid syndrome, 606
    for celiac disease, 645
    for somatostatinoma syndrome, 607
    neutropenic enterocolitis in, 690
Chlamydia trachomatis infections, 682
Cholestyramine
    for functional diarrhea, 633
    for inflammatory bowel disease, 667
    for microscopic colitis, 657
Chronic diarrhea
    circulating agents causing, **603–610**
    colorectal histology and histopathology in, **561–580**
    functional, **629–637**
    gut microbiota and, **581–602**
    in carbohydrate malabsorption, **611–627,** 660–662
    in celiac disease, **639–650**
    in immunocompromise, **677–701**
    in inflammatory bowel diseases. *See* Inflammatory bowel disease.
    stool analysis for. *See* Stool analysis.
Chronic granulomatous disease, 692
Cidofovir, for cytomegalovirus infections, 686
Ciprofloxacin
    for bacterial overgrowth, 667
    for cyclosporiasis, 681
    for inflammatory bowel disease, 592, 594–595
    for irritable bowel syndrome, 592–593
Circulating agents, diarrhea caused by, **603–610**
    endocrine diarrheal syndrome, 604–605
    hyperthyroidism, 607
    malignant carcinoid syndrome, 605–606
    mastocytosis, 607
    pancreatic tumors, 608
    somatostatinoma syndrome, 607
    thyroid carcinoma, 607
    Zollinger-Ellison syndrome, 606–607
Clarithromycin
    for inflammatory bowel disease, 592
    for mycobacterial infections, 683

Clindamycin, carbohydrate metabolism and, 614
Clofazimine, for inflammatory bowel disease, 592
Clonidine, for functional diarrhea, 634
Clostridium difficile infections
    in immunocompromise, 683–684
    in inflammatory bowel disease, 664
    treatment of, 667–668
Codeine
    for functional diarrhea, 631–632
    for inflammatory bowel disease, 668
Colestipol, for inflammatory bowel disease, 667
Colitis. *See also* Enterocolitis.
    collagenous, 564–567
    cord, 690
    diverticular disease-associated, 574, 576
    indeterminate, 573
    lymphocytic, 564–567
    microscopic, 652–658
        histopathology of, 564–568
        in celiac disease, 644
    of uncertain type, 573
    pseudomembranous collagenous, 568
    ulcerative. *See* Ulcerative colitis.
Collagenous colitis, 564–567
Colon, resection of
    carbohydrate malabsorption in, 617
    diarrhea after, 663–664
Colonoscopy
    for cytomegalovirus infections, 685
    for functional diarrhea, 630–631
    for microscopic colitis, 566–567, 655
Colorectal histopathology, **561–580**
    in inflammatory bowel disease, 570–576
    in mast cell enterocolitis, 568–569
    in microscopic colitis, 564–568
    versus normal histology, 562–564
Common variable immunodeficiency, 691–692
Computed tomography, for inflammatory bowel disease, 666
Congenital immunodeficiency syndromes, 691–692
Cord colitis syndrome, 690
Crohn disease, 658–665
    diagnosis of, 573–576
    gut microbiota alterations in, 583
    histopathology of, 570–572
    treatment of, 590–592, 594–595
    versus ulcerative colitis, 573–576
Cryptal lymphocytic coloproctitis, 568
Cryptosporidiosis, 680
Crypts
    in colorectal mucosa, 562–563
    in inflammatory bowel disease, 570–571

Culture, for gut microbiota, 584
Cyclosporiasis, 681
Cyclosporine, for graft-versus-host disease, 689
Cytomegalovirus infections, 685–686

D

Dairy products, intolerance of, 618–619, 621, 662
Desipramine, for functional diarrhea, 632
Diet
    for celiac disease, 639–640, 643–644
    for functional diarrhea, 631
DiGeorge syndrome, 692
Diphenoxylate
    for functional diarrhea, 631–632
    for inflammatory bowel disease, 667–668
Disaccharidase deficiencies, 620–621
Diverticular disease-associated colitis, 574, 576
Drugs, diarrhea induced by
    in immunocompromise, 688, 690–691
    in inflammatory bowel disease, 664–665

E

Electron microscopy, for microsporidiosis, 687
Encephalitozoon intestinalis infections, 687
Endocrine diarrheal syndrome, 604–605
Endomysial antibody, in celiac disease, 642
Enkephalinase inhibitors, for functional diarrhea, 632–633
Enterocolitis
    mast cell, 568–569
    neutropenic, 690
Enterocytozoon bieneusi infections, 687
Enteropathy
    gluten. See Celiac disease.
    idiopathic AIDS, 687–688
Enzyme immunoassays, for Clostridium difficile, 684
Epithelial lymphocytosis, 568
Escherichia coli Nissle, for inflammatory bowel disease, 590–591
Ethambutol, for mycobacterial infections, 683
Everolimus, for VIPoma syndrome, 605

F

Fat malabsorption, 660–661
Fiber, for functional diarrhea, 633
Fidaxomicin, for Clostridium difficile infections, 684
Fistulas, in inflammatory bowel disease, 662–663
Fluid therapy
    for cryptosporidiosis, 680
    for norovirus infections, 686

Fluoroquinolones
    for cord colitis syndrome, 690
    for mycobacterial infections, 683
5-Fluorouracil, for VIPoma syndrome, 605
Foscarnet, for cytomegalovirus infections, 685–686
Fructose malabsorption, 619–621
Functional diarrhea, **629–637**
    definition of, 629–630
    diagnosis of, 630–631
    epidemiology of, 630
    pathophysiology of, 631
    treatment of, 631–634
Fungal infections, 686–687

G

Galacto-oligosaccharide, for inflammatory bowel disease, 590
Galactose malabsorption, 620–621
Ganciclovir, for cytomegalovirus infections, 685–686
Gas production, 613–614, 618–619
Gastric bypass, carbohydrate malabsorption in, 617–618
Gastritis, in inflammatory bowel disease, 572
Gastrocolic fistulas, in inflammatory bowel disease, 662
Gastronomes, in Zollinger-Ellison syndrome, 607
Genetic factors
    in fructose malabsorption, 620
    in lactose malabsorption, 618–619, 621–622
Glucagonoma syndrome, 608
Glucose breath test, for gut microbiota evaluation, 584
Glucose-galastose malabsorption, 620–621
Gluten enteropathy. *See* Celiac disease.
Goblet cells, histology of, 562
Graft-versus-host disease, 688–691
Granulomatous inflammation, in microscopic colitis, 568
Gum agar, for functional diarrhea, 633
Gut microbiota, **581–602**
    homeostasis disturbances in, 582–584
    modulation of
        factors affecting, 585–587
        for chronic diarrhea, 587–595
    mucosal barrier and, 582
    overgrowth of. *See* Bacterial overgrowth.
    physiology of, 582
    studies of, 584–585

H

Histopathology, colorectal. *See* Colorectal histopathology.
HIV enteropathy, 687–688
Human immunodeficiency virus infections, diarrhea in, 679, 687–688
Human leukocyte antigens, in celiac disease, 642

Hydrogen breath test
   applications of, 620
   for bacterial overgrowth syndrome, 663
   for fructose malabsorption, 620
   for gut microbiota evaluation, 584
   for inflammatory bowel disease, 666
5-Hydroxyindoleacetic acid, in carcinoid syndrome, 606
5-Hydroxytryptophan inhibitors, for functional diarrhea, 632
Hyperinfection, in strongyloidiasis, 681
Hyperthyroidism, 607
Hypochlorhydria, in VIPoma syndrome, 604–605
Hypogammaglobulinemic sprue, 691
Hypolactasia, 618–619

I

Idiopathic AIDS enteropathy, 687–688
Ileocolonosopy, for inflammatory bowel disease, 666
Ileosigmoid fistulas, in inflammatory bowel disease, 662
Immune dysregulation–polyendocrinopathy–enteropathy–X-linked syndrome, 692
Immunocompromise, diarrhea in, **677–701**
   drug-induced, 688, 690–691
   in congenital immunodeficiency, 691—692
   infectious
      agents causing, *677–679*
      bacterial, 681–684
      fungal, 686–687
      in HIV infections, 679, 687–688
      parasitic, 680–681
      viral, 684–686
   noninfectious, 678, 687–688
   transplant-related, 688–690
Immunoglobulin A deficiency, 691
Indeterminate colitis, 573
Infections
   gut microbiota alterations in, 583
   in immunocompromise. *See* Immunocompromise.
Inflammatory bowel disease, **651–675**. *See also* Crohn disease; Ulcerative colitis.
   causes of, 660–665
   diagnosis of, 573–576
   gut microbiota alterations in, 583
   histopathology of, 570–572
   microscopic colitis, 652–658
   pathophysiology of, 659–660
   treatment of, 590–592, 594–595, 667–668
   unclassified, 573
   versus irritable bowel syndrome, 665
   versus normal intestinal fluid transport, 652
Infliximab
   for graft-versus-host disease, 689
   for microscopic colitis, 658
Intraepithelial lymphocytes, in microscopic colitis, 565

Intraluminal agents, for functional diarrhea, 633–634
Irritable bowel syndrome, 665
    gut microbiota alterations in, 583–584
    treatment of, 587–588, 592–593
Isosporiasis, 681
Ispaghula husk, for functional diarrhea, 633
Itraconazole, for histoplasmosis, 687
Ivermectin, for strongyloidiasis, 681

L

Lactase deficiency, 618–619
Lactic acid, formation of, in carbohydrate metabolism, 612–613
Lactobacillus acidophilus
    for functional diarrhea, 633
    for irritable bowel syndrome, 587–588
Lactobacillus bulgaricus, for antibiotic-associated diarrhea, 590
Lactobacillus casei, for antibiotic-associated diarrhea, 590
Lactobacillus GG
    for antibiotic-associated diarrhea, 589–590
    for inflammatory bowel disease, 590–591
    for irritable bowel syndrome, 587
Lactobacillus helviticus, for irritable bowel syndrome, 587–588
Lactobacillus plantarum, for irritable bowel syndrome, 587–588
Lactobacillus reuteri, for antibiotic-associated diarrhea, 589–590
Lactobacillus rhamnosus
    for antibiotic-associated diarrhea, 589
    for irritable bowel syndrome, 587–588
Lactose breath test, 619
Lactose malabsorption, 618–619, 621, 631, 662
Lactulose
    colonic transit and, 616
    ingestion of, stool analysis in, 622
Lactulose hydrogen breath test, for gut microbiota evaluation, 584
Lamina propria
    histology of, 564
    in inflammatory bowel disease, 570
Laxatives, osmotic, 556
Levofloxacin, for mycobacterial infections, 683
Lidamidine, for functional diarrhea, 634
Loperamide
    for functional diarrhea, 631–632
    for inflammatory bowel disease, 667–668
    for microscopic colitis, 655
Lymphocytic colitis, 564–567
Lymphoma, T-cell, in celiac disease, 644–645

M

Magnesium-induced diarrhea, diagnosis of, 547
Magnetic resonance imaging, for inflammatory bowel disease, 666

Malabsorption, carbohydrate. *See* Carbohydrate malabsorption.
Malignant carcinoid syndrome, 605–606
Mast cells, in colorectal mucosa, 563–564
Mastocytosis, 568–569, 607
Medullary carcinoma, thyroid, 607
6-Mercaptopurine, for microscopic colitis, 657–658
Mesalamine, for inflammatory bowel disease, 591
Mesalazine
    for inflammatory bowel disease, 594
    for microscopic colitis, 657
Metastasis
    from carcinoid tumors, 605–606
    from VIPoma syndrome, 605
Methotrexate, for microscopic colitis, 657–658
Methylcellulose, for inflammatory bowel disease, 668
Methylprednisolone
    for graft-versus-host disease, 689
    for inflammatory bowel disease, 594
Metronidazole
    carbohydrate metabolism and, 615
    for bacterial overgrowth, 592–593, 667
    for *Clostridium difficile* infections, 667, 684
    for cord colitis syndrome, 690
    for inflammatory bowel disease, 592,
        594–595
    for irritable bowel syndrome, 592–593
Microflora. *See* Gut microbiota.
Microscopic colitis, 652–658
    atypical, 567–568
    causes of, 653–654
    classification of, 568
    clinical presentation of, 654–655
    diagnosis of, 655
    differential diagnosis of, 656
    epidemiology of, 653
    histopathology of, 564–568
    history of, 652–653
    in celiac disease, 644
    pathophysiology of, 654
    paucicellular, 568
    treatment of, 655, 657–658
    variants of, 567–568
Microsporidiosis, 687
Morphine
    for functional diarrhea, 631
    for inflammatory bowel disease, 668
Moxifloxacin, for mycobacterial infections, 683
Multiple endocrine neoplasia, 607
Mycobacterial infections, 682–683
Mycophenolate mofetil, diarrhea induced by, 690–691

N

Neomycin, for irritable bowel syndrome, 592
Neuroendocrine neoplasia, 605–606
Neutropenic enterocolitis, 690
Nitazoxanide, for cryptosporidiosis, 680
Norovirus infections, 686
Nutritional support, for norovirus infections, 686

O

Octreotide, for functional diarrhea, 634
Opioid agonists, for functional diarrhea, 631–632
Opium, for inflammatory bowel disease, 668
Organic acids, formation of, in carbohydrate metabolism, 612–614
Ornidazol, for inflammatory bowel disease, 595
Osmotic activity, organic acids and, 612–613
Osmotic diarrhea, versus secretory diarrhea, 544

P

Pancreas, neuroendocrine tumors of, 608
Pancreatic cholera syndrome, 604–605
Pancreatic disease, carbohydrate malabsorption in, 617
Pancreatic polypeptide, tumors producing, 608
Paneth cells, histology of, 562
Parasitic infections, 680–681
Parenteral nutrition, for norovirus infections, 686
Paucicellular microscopic colitis, 568
Peptic ulcer disease, in Zollinger-Ellison syndrome, 606–607
Plasma cells, in colorectal mucosa, 563
Polycarbophil, for inflammatory bowel disease, 668
Polyethylene glycol, colonic transit and, 616
Pouchitis, 590, 594–595
Prebiotics, gut microbiota alterations by, 585–586
Precursor cells, in colorectal mucosa, 562–563
Prednisolone
    for graft-versus-host disease, 689
    for microscopic colitis, 657
Proabsorptive drugs, for functional diarrhea, 634
Probiotics
    for antibiotic-associated diarrhea, 587, 589–590
    for functional diarrhea, 633
    for inflammatory bowel disease, 590–591
    for irritable bowel syndrome, 587–588
    gut microbiota alterations by, 585–586
Propionate, formation of, in carbohydrate metabolism, 612–613
Propionibacterium freudenreichii, for irritable bowel syndrome, 587–588
Protease inhibitors, diarrhea induced by, 688
Proton pump inhibitors, for Zollinger-Ellison syndrome, 607
Pseudomembranous collagenous colitis, 568

Pseudopancreatic cholera, 605
Psyllium
    for functional diarrhea, 633
    for inflammatory bowel disease, 668

R

Racecadotril, for functional diarrhea, 632–633
Ramosetron, for functional diarrhea, 632
Rifabutin, for mycobacterial infections, 683
Rifaximin
    for bacterial overgrowth, 592–593, 667
    for *Clostridium difficile* infections, 684
    for irritable bowel syndrome, 592–593
    gut microbiota alterations by, 587
RNA analysis, for gut microbiota, 584–585
Rome III Criteria, functional diarrhea definition of, 629–630
Roux-en-Y gastric bypass, carbohydrate malabsorption in, 617–618

S

Saccharomyces boulardii
    for antibiotic-associated diarrhea, 587–589
    for inflammatory bowel disease, 590–591
    for irritable bowel syndrome, 587
Salmonella infections, 682
Secretin test, for Zollinger-Ellison syndrome, 607
Secretinomas, 608
Secretory diarrhea, versus osmotic diarrhea, 544
Segmental colitis associated with diverticulosis, 574, 576
Serologic tests, for celiac disease, 642
Severe combined immunodeficiency, 692
Sigmoidoscopy, for microscopic colitis, 566–567, 655
Small bowel capsule endoscopy, for inflammatory bowel disease, 666
Small intestine
    biopsy of, in celiac disease, 642–643
    resection of
        carbohydrate malabsorption in, 617
        diarrhea after, 663–664
Somatostatin analogs, for functional diarrhea, 634
Somatostatinoma syndrome, 607
Sorbitol, ingestion of, stool analysis in, 622
Stains, for microsporidiosis, 687
Starch, metabolism of, 613–614
Steatorrhea
    diagnosis of, 542–544, 555
    in inflammatory bowel disease, 661, 666–667
    in Zollinger-Ellison syndrome, 607
Stem cell transplantation, 688–691
Stool analysis
    diagnostic value of, **539–560**
    for carbohydrate malabsorption, 622

Stool (*continued*)
　　for *Chlamydia trachomatis* infections, 682
　　for cryptosporidiosis, 680
　　for histoplasmosis, 686
　　for inflammatory bowel disease, 666
　　for strongyloidiasis, 681
Stool transplantation, for *Clostridium difficile* infections, 684
Streptococcus faecium, for irritable bowel syndrome, 587
Streptococcus thermophilus, for antibiotic-associated diarrhea, 590
Streptozocin
　　for somatostatinoma syndrome, 607
　　for VIPoma syndrome, 605
Stress, functional diarrhea in, 631
Strongyloidiasis, 680–681
Sucrase-isomaltase deficiency, 620

T

T cells, in celiac disease, 644–645
Tetracyclines
　　for bacterial overgrowth, 667
　　for inflammatory bowel disease, 595
Thiabendazole, for strongyloidiasis, 681
Thyroid, medullary carcinoma of, 607
Tinidazole, for inflammatory bowel disease, 594
Tissue transglutaminase, in celiac disease, 642
Toll-like receptors, gut microbiota interactions with, 582
Toxins, *Clostridium difficile,* 683–684
Transfusions, graft-versus-host disease in, 690
Transit, colonic
　　carbohydrate metabolism and, 615–616
　　in HIV infection, 688
　　inhibitors of, for functional diarrhea, 631–633
Transplantation, solid organ and stem cell, 688–691
Trehalase deficiency, 620
Tricyclic antidepressants, for functional diarrhea, 632
Trimethoprim-sulfamethoxazole
　　for bacterial overgrowth, 667
　　for cyclosporiasis, 681
Tuberculosis, 682–683
Tumor necrosis factor inhibitors, for microscopic colitis, 658

U

Ulcerative colitis, 658–665
　　diagnosis of, 573–576
　　gut microbiota alterations in, 583
　　histopathology of, 570–572
　　treatment of, 590–592, 594–595
　　versus Crohn disease, 573–576
Ulcerative rectocolitis, in *Chlamydia trachomatis* infections, 682

V

Vancomycin, for *Clostridium difficile* infections, 667, 684
Vangancyclovir, for cytomegalovirus infections, 685
Verner-Morrison syndrome, 604–605
Villous atrophy
   carbohydrate malabsorption in, 617
   in celiac disease, 642–643
VIPoma syndrome, 604–605
Viral infections, 684–686
VSL#3 probiotic mixture
   for inflammatory bowel disease, 590–591
   for irritable bowel syndrome, 587–588

W

Water diarrhea hypokalemia hypochlorhydria syndrome, 604–605

X

X-linked infantile agammaglobulinemia, 692

Z

Zollinger-Ellison syndrome, 606–607

Moving?

Make sure your subscription moves with you!

To notify us of your new address, find your **Clinics Account Number** (located on your mailing label above your name), and contact customer service at:

Email: journalscustomerservice-usa@elsevier.com

800-654-2452 (subscribers in the U.S. & Canada)
314-447-8871 (subscribers outside of the U.S. & Canada)

Fax number: 314-447-8029

Elsevier Health Sciences Division
Subscription Customer Service
3251 Riverport Lane
Maryland Heights, MO 63043

*To ensure uninterrupted delivery of your subscription, please notify us at least 4 weeks in advance of move.

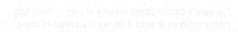

Printed and bound by CPI Group (UK) Ltd, Croydon, CR0 4YY

03/10/2024

01040458-0015